Increasing Patient Satisfaction With Statistical Correlation

A Step-by-Step Guide to the JCAHO's Staffing Effectiveness Standards

Cynthia Barnard, MBA, CPHQ

Samuel F. Hohmann, PhD, MSHSM

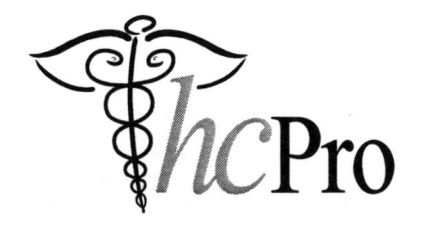

hcPro

Increasing Patient Satisfaction With Statistical Correlation: A Step-by-Step Guide to the JCAHO's Staffing Effectiveness Standards is published by HCPro, Inc.

Copyright 2003 by HCPro, Inc.

All rights reserved. Printed in the United States of America.   5   4   3   2   1

ISBN 1-57839-268-3

No part of this publication may be reproduced, in any form or by any means, without prior written consent of HCPro or the Copyright Clearance Center (978/750-8400). Please notify us immediately if you have received an unauthorized copy.

HCPro provides information resources for the health care industry.

HCPro is not affiliated in any way with the Joint Commission on Accreditation of Healthcare Organizations, which owns the JCAHO trademark.

Cynthia Barnard, MBA, CPHQ, Co-author
Samuel F. Hohmann, PhD, MSHSM, Co-author
Molly Hall, Managing Editor
Matthew Cann, Group Publisher
Jean St. Pierre, Creative Director
Mike Mirabello, Senior Graphic Artist
Matthew Sharpe, Graphic Artist
Jacqueline Diehl Singer, Layout Artist
Paul Singer, Layout Artist
Steven DeGrappo, Cover Designer
Suzanne Perney, Publisher

Advice given is general. Readers should consult professional counsel for specific legal, ethical, or clinical questions.

Arrangements can be made for quantity discounts. For more information, contact:

HCPro
P.O. Box 1168
Marblehead, MA 01945
Telephone: 800/650-6787 or 781/639-1872
Fax: 781/639-2982
E-mail: customerservice@hcpro.com

Visit HCPro at its World Wide Web sites:
www.hcmarketplace.com, www.hcpro.com, and *www.accreditinfo.com*

Contents

About the Authors v

Preface vi

Introduction ix

Section I: Background 1

    Patient satisfaction as a meaningful outcome of care 3

    Defining patient satisfaction 6

    The connection between patient satisfaction and staffing 10

    Why staffing effectiveness? 12

    The relationship of patient satisfaction to staffing effectiveness 13

    The emergence of the staffing effectiveness standards 13

Section II: The Standards 15

    Description of the standards 17

    Getting started 20

Section III: Step-by-Step Guide to Meeting the Staffing Effectiveness Standards 27

    Choosing your indicators 29

    Collecting and using your data 41

    Recording your data 48

Contents

    Analyzing your data 60

    Presenting your data 102

Conclusion: What to Do Next 121

    What if you find a correlation 123

    What is a staffing plan? 125

    Final steps 128

    Final considerations 132

Appendix A: Glossary 133

Appendix B: Tools 143

About the Authors

Cynthia Barnard, MBA, CPHQ, is Director, Quality Strategies, at Northwestern Memorial Hospital, affiliated with Northwestern University Feinberg School of Medicine. She is responsible for the patient safety program's quality improvement initiatives, including patient satisfaction measurement, accreditation, and licensure compliance, and support of medical ethics. Prior roles at Northwestern and elsewhere have included a decade in quality improvement, direction of the hospital safety program, seven years directing medical staff affairs and clinical research, and 10 years developing and consulting on health care information systems for operational support and strategic planning and analysis. Cynthia also planned, built, and managed the hospital's day care center. She holds a master's degree in management from Northwestern University's Kellogg School of Management, a bachelor's degree in psychology, magna cum laude, from Bryn Mawr College, and a Certified Professional in Healthcare Quality designation from the National Association for Healthcare Quality. She is the co-author of the book *Performance Improvement: Winning Strategies for Quality and JCAHO Compliance*, published by HCPro (now in its second edition), which won the NAHQ's 2000 award for publication excellence.

Samuel F. Hohmann, PhD, MSHSM, has over 15 years of health care experience working in statistical research, quality improvement, and risk management. He is currently the senior research specialist in information architecture for the University HealthSystem Consortium (UHC). Prior to joining UHC, he was the director of integrated advanced information management systems (IAIMS) and quality improvement systems (QIS) at the Center for Clinical Effectiveness (CCE), Loyola University Health System. Sam previously served as vice president of research and statistics at QuadraMed Corporation. In his current role, Sam is responsible for producing Periodic Member Assessments, in which operational and clinical performance improvement opportunities are identified, as well as for conducting administrative and research data analysis in support of the corporate information architecture mission and goals of the University HealthSystem Consortium. Sam has also held positions with MMI Companies, Inc., as executive director of its Institute for Healthcare Risk Management Studies and as assistant vice president.

Preface

The most critical trends facing hospitals and health care providers in the first decade of the 21st century all revolve around how we use and support our staffs to deliver safe and effective care. Consider the concerns reflected on the agenda of every health care leader:

- There is a national **shortage of health care workers** in key professions, such as nursing, pharmacy, radiography, and anesthesiology.
- Increasing evidence shows that **appropriate staffing has a measurable impact on clinical outcomes.**
- The question of appropriate staffing is rapidly becoming the focus of many **health care unions,** which are addressing the issue both by negotiating contracts and lobbying for state legislation to mandate staffing ratios.
- The development of data supporting **"evidence-based" medical practice** offers a model for systematic and predictable delivery of the right care by the right staff at the right time.
- **Patient confidence** in the health care system is at a crisis level, which is well documented in studies reporting an overall lack of trust in the system, as well as beliefs that medical error is common and that health care providers do not disclose information about errors accurately.
- Payer and regulatory confidence in providers is now linked to a demand for **public accountability through performance measures,** whether from the Joint Commission for the Accreditation of Healthcare Organizations (JCAHO), the Centers for Medicare and Medicaid Services (CMS), or employer organizations, such as Leapfrog Group.
- Responding to these trends, CMS is designing and implementing a national patient satisfaction survey with a public release of results planned for late 2004 or 2005.

Successful organizations are moving ahead rapidly to ensure that they understand and optimize the relationship between effective staffing and patient outcomes. This critical success factor finds its way into the accreditation standards for hospitals via the JCAHO requirement for staffing effectiveness, analysis, and improvement.

Achieving compliance with this new standard is not merely part of a routine effort to achieve accred-

Preface

itation. If designed properly, compliance efforts can be secondary to **fundamental improvement of patient satisfaction outcomes.**

Effective and meaningful data collection and management is, in and of itself, a difficult subject in health care, where it is challenging to find reliable measures in the face of complexity and variability among patients.

As with many JCAHO standards, the staffing effectiveness standards are challenging because they are not prescriptive, meaning it's up to you to define your process. You can collect, analyze, and use the data in whatever manner you choose—as long as you can provide reasoning for why you selected a certain method and can demonstrate your attempt to correlate outcomes.

The trick to compliance isn't just putting data on paper but being able to articulate why and how you selected these measures, how you derived results and what you did with them, and how your staff are engaging with the effort continuously. In order to achieve full compliance, you will need to ensure that your governing body, senior management, and staff can describe what "staffing effectiveness" means in your organization.

And of course, as a leader in your organization, you are well aware that compliance should be a *byproduct* of excellent practice and programs. In other words, your goals are to improve care and service to your patients, support your staff effectively, and achieve compliance as a part of that process. You want to make a difference for patient care—not simply score compliance.

To this end, we will take you through a step-by-step process of selecting your indicators, collecting data, analyzing relationships, and presenting results. We will prepare you not only to meet the standard but also to understand and recognize the potential patient satisfaction benefits. We will do this by demonstrating tools and using real examples throughout the book. **Regardless of the specific indicators you select, you should be able to adapt or modify our examples to meet the individual needs of your facility.**

We designed this book to demonstrate easy-to-use methods for staffing effectiveness and standards compliance. Our methods will help you conduct statistical analysis effectively with a basic understanding of data management analysis methods. Our companion Excel spreadsheet will enable you to record data, make statistical calculations automatically, and produce graphic presentations of your results. Using that spreadsheet as a tool, we will walk you through the steps of understanding the JCAHO staffing standards, selecting the indicators to evaluate, and establishing a staffing plan based on your data.

Preface

The workbook contains three primary sections:

- The connection between patient satisfaction and staffing
- Staffing effectiveness overview
- A how-to guide for data collection, analysis, and presentation

In each of these sections you will find tools, graphs, and directions to ensure your ability to demonstrate your use of data for compliance with the staffing standards and to enhance patient satisfaction. We also include information to assist you in educating your staff, management, and leaders on the interplay between patient satisfaction and staffing effectiveness.

Whether you've already selected your indicators or you're just starting out, we know you will find ***Increasing Patient Satisfaction With Statistical Correlation: A Step-by-Step Guide to the JCAHO's Staffing Effectiveness Standards*** a useful tool in enhancing patient satisfaction and ensuring staffing effectiveness.

Introduction

The American health care delivery system is working to respond to increasing pressure for public accountability for effective, safe, and high quality care, in an era of shortages of health care workers in key areas such as nursing, pharmacy, and radiology. A core strategy is to ensure that you can quantify adequate staffing (numbers and mix) to achieve desired outcomes of care.

Most hospitals are now facing slim revenue margins, or even losses, on operations. Limited resources, coupled with cyclical staff shortages, make the task of allocating effective staff even more challenging.

The public focus on accountability and consumerism has also been reflected in an increasing demand for measurement of the "patient experience" of care. The most dramatic expression of this change is in the development of the new Medicare "H-CAHPS" survey of patient satisfaction in hospitals.

In 2002, Medicare launched a project under the direction of the federal Agency for Healthcare Research and Quality (AHRQ, www.ahrq.gov) to develop a valid and reliable national tool to measure the patient experience. The data that will be assembled from this effort is explicitly intended for dissemination, consistent with the aims expressed in the federally sponsored report, *Envisioning the National Health Care Quality Report* (National Academies Press, 2001).

Thus, it is a given that patient satisfaction data specific to health care organizations will be collected and published. The specifics of how this will occur will continue to evolve; however, every hospital and health delivery system should be working actively to ensure that the dynamics of patient satisfaction are understood thoroughly and that the connection with staffing is addressed comprehensively.

In short, patient satisfaction and quality of care depend on appropriate staffing decisions and the successful implementation of those decisions. Public disclosure of data reflecting your performance on these measures is part of the inevitable strategic present and future of every health care organization.

Introduction

Partly in recognition of these developing trends, the JCAHO released a standard known as "staffing effectiveness," which became effective for hospitals in July 2002, with other programs following thereafter (the standard becomes effective for long-term care and assisted-living facilities in January 2004).

This standard requires organizations to collect, analyze, measure, and use data to evaluate the effect of staffing on patient outcomes. The purpose of this process is to integrate human resources factors (such as nursing hours) and clinical patient outcomes data (such as mortality, complications, or patient complaints) to establish parameters for effective staffing and to enhance patient outcomes.

The JCAHO's standard requires hospitals to

- develop a hypothesis, theory, or exploratory plan to evaluate the effect of at least two different measures of staffing on at least two different measures of outcome (there will be two pairs of measures, each of which contains a single staffing indicator and a single clinical or service performance measure)

- identify and define two different human resources (HR) screening measures for data collection and use (and determine which care providers will be included in the HR indicators)

- identify and define at least two different clinical screening measures for data collection and use (and identify target or expected performance on these outcomes)

- demonstrate that leadership has developed a rationale for selection and testing of the relationship of these measures.

- articulate and plan a mechanism for data collection, measurement, and analysis

- explore and identify variations in the data and potential causes of variation in the targeted outcomes

- use collected data to evaluate the effectiveness of staffing decisions in achieving targeted patient outcomes

- use the relationships that have been evaluated to assess current staffing plans, adjust them, and implement revised staffing, where indicated

- define what, when, and how to report to leadership the effectiveness of staffing and any actions taken to improve staffing

Introduction

Although the JCAHO standard clearly defines a goal that requires measurement, the manner and method of this measurement is left up to the organization. While measurement has been part of many JCAHO standards for more than a decade, the staffing effectiveness standard requires an additional degree of sophistication and complexity. Staffing effectiveness is based on the *relationship* among measures (people measures and clinical measures) and may require an integration of leaders and thought processes that have not been integrated previously. In many settings, it is easy for clinical leaders to believe that staffing affects outcomes but difficult for them to articulate this in a quantitative or demonstrable way. And it may be a new, or even foreign, concept for HR professionals to accept accountability for clinical outcomes associated with the staffing plans and decisions that they make.

For the individual or team tagged with coordinating responsibility for this effort, selecting the right approach in your hospital may not be easy—especially while balancing a multitude of other job-related functions. In many hospitals, it won't be a statistician who is responsible for designing and implementing a data collection strategy; it may be the performance (quality) improvement department or the JCAHO survey coordinator who is responsible—regardless of his or her experience with statistics. Our goal is to simplify this process by providing clear measurement techniques and reducing the fear that many people experience when implementing statistical control measures.

This book is designed to walk even the most inexperienced of data analyzers through the process of selecting the required two indicators (we'll focus on patient satisfaction and nursing hours) and collecting, aggregating, and analyzing data for those indicators. **Regardless of the indicators you select, you should be able to adapt or modify our examples to meet the particular needs of your facility.**

We'll also show you some common mistakes in the process so that you can avoid them. Perhaps most important, we'll show you what to do with the data once you've got it, and how to use it to demonstrate whether there is a correlation between your indicators. We will do more than just show you how to meet JCAHO standards; we'll show you how data can improve patient satisfaction through the use of effective staffing plans.

Meeting JCAHO standards is important for any accredited organization. Meeting the needs of every patient for a high quality, satisfying, safe, and effective outcome is even more important. By employing the staffing effectiveness standards with valid and reliable data and a solid management plan, you can accomplish both goals.

Section I
Background

Section I: Background

Patient satisfaction as a meaningful outcome of care

Research literature suggests that

- patients are capable of evaluating many aspects of the technical quality of care

- meeting patients' needs for an overall satisfactory experience improves their compliance with treatment recommendations and, therefore, clinical outcomes

- a positive relationship with health care providers reduces litigation

- there is a close relationship between patient and employee satisfaction (Satisfied employees provide care that better meets patients' needs, and a satisfied patient population provides a more positive work environment)[1]

In addition, the "business case" for patient satisfaction emerges from the value of a health care provider's reputation and the evident truth that "word of mouth" is a powerful driver of referrals.

JCAHO standards for accreditation have required some attention to the patient's and family's perception of care for more than a decade, and most hospitals have responded by implementing some sort of patient survey to collect systematic data regarding the patient's experience. (See JCAHO standard

---

[1] For a useful overview of the literature on this subject, consult Irwin Press, *Patient Satisfaction: Defining, Measuring, and Improving the Experience of Care* (Health Administrative Press,. 2002).

Section I: Background

PI.3.1: *"Organizations are required to collect data about the needs, expectations, and satisfaction of individuals and organizations served... their perceptions of how well the organization meets these needs and expectations."*)

Nonetheless, in contrast to more traditional measures of clinical outcomes, patient satisfaction measures have faced an uphill battle as a useful indicator of health care delivery system performance.

Early community-based initiatives in Cleveland, Rochester (NY), and elsewhere encountered resistance from clinicians and health care administrators, who argued that the data were subjective, not valid or reliable. Most of these local experiments have been discontinued, although individual payers still conduct surveys in some markets.

Even the largest payer-employer consortia driving regional or national measurement in their markets (Washington Business Group on Health, Midwest Business Group on Health, Leapfrog Group, etc.) have tended to downplay the role of patient satisfaction measurement in their efforts to collect and publish data for quality improvement and accountability.

This historical pattern, however, is undergoing a dramatic change. A new national effort seeks to measure and publish data on patients' experience of care, specifically to help patients select a provider of care—and, secondarily, to help providers to improve.

A nationally validated tool for the "Consumer Assessment of Health Plans" (CAHPS) was developed in 1995 by a consortium coordinated by a federal agency (now titled the Agency for Healthcare Research and Quality [AHRQ], *www.ahrq.gov*). This tool is now commonly used among many employers, payers, and plans.[2]

Later, the President's Advisory Commission on Consumer Protection and Quality in the Health Care Industry (1998) articulated a specific goal of publishing quality data to assist the industry to improve, and consumers to make informed choices.[3]

---

[2] Consumer Assessment of Health Plans (CAHPS®): Fact Sheet. AHRQ Publication No. 00-PO47, April 2000. Agency for Healthcare Research and Policy, Rockville, MD. *http://www.ahrg.gov/qual/cahpfact.htm*

[3] President's Advisory Commission on Consumer Protection and Quality in the Health Care Industry, July 1998, at *http://www.hcqualitycommission.gov/final/execsum.html*

"A key element of improving health care quality is the Nation's ability to measure the quality of care and provide easily understood, comparable information on the performance of the industry. Advances in quality measurement and reporting have enabled us to determine the flaws in the current system. But the absence of a systematic approach to quality measurement has hampered the health care industry's ability to track and sustain quality improvement."

Section I: Background

A subsequent phase of the patient survey work for managed care plans was launched by Centers for Medicare and Medicaid Services, through AHRQ, to develop a similar survey or assessment tool for use related to hospital experiences. CMS confirmed that the agency seeks to develop a "hospital patient survey as a means of obtaining comparative information for consumers who need to select a hospital and as a way of encouraging accountability of hospitals for the care they provide. The ultimate goal of this effort, both for AHRQ and CMS, is high quality care for hospital patients."[4]

These initiatives are consistent with an overarching federal effort to improve and open to public review all aspects of patient care. Two recent federal research reports establish the framework.

In 2001, the Institute of Medicine (IOM) released its report, *Crossing the Quality Chasm: A New Health System for the 21st Century*.[5] In this report, the IOM listed six goals for health care. Health care should be

- safe—by avoiding injuries

- effective

- patient centered

- timely

- equitable

- efficient

A subsequent report by the Committee on Enhancing Federal Healthcare Quality Programs, *Leadership by Example*,[6] addresses the need to establish a government leadership role in improving health care quality. This report focuses on the need for a strong quality infrastructure consisting of three components:

---

[4] www.ahcpr.gov/qual/cahps/hcahpstrans.htm
[5] Committee on Quality of Health Care in America, IOM. *Crossing the Quality Chasm: A New Health System for the 21st Century* (National Academies Press, 2001).
[6] Committee on Enhancing Federal Healthcare Quality Programs, Janet M. Corrigan, Jill Eden, and Barbara M. Smith, Editors. *Leadership by Example: Coordinating Government Roles in Improving Health Care Quality*. (National Academies Press, 2002).

Section I: Background

- Standardized performance measures in government programs, including patient perception measures explicitly

- Financial support to facilitate the development of technology infrastructures

- Government programs making quality reports available in the public domain

Defining patient satisfaction

Measurement of patient satisfaction or perceptions of care is not only the "right thing to do" as part of a health care provider's mission. It is also important for clinical benefit, marketing and referrals, risk management, accreditation, employee satisfaction, and future public accountability.

There are, however, a number of approaches to defining satisfaction, and each organization will select an approach (or, sometimes, a set of approaches) that meets the needs of the provider.

Decision 1: What do we mean by "satisfaction"?
    Option 1: Patient provides a **rating** of how he or she feels that you performed on several important aspects of care.
    Option 2: Patient provides feedback on actual **experience**: how consistently you delivered specific behaviors.
    Option 3: You **count** or evaluate the number of specific **complaints** or "defects" in care.

Decision 2: How will you find out what your patients think?
Let's consider each of these in turn.

First, Decision 1: What do we mean by "satisfaction"? There are three primary approaches to the measurement of patient satisfaction.

Option 1: Ratings

Traditional patient satisfaction surveys evaluate the patient's feelings or perceptions about aspects of care and service. Patients are invited to rate items such as the "friendliness of the nurse" or the "helpfulness of discharge information." Typically, a response scale is used, e.g. "very poor, poor, fair, good, very good." Some form of algorithm is then used to integrate the results into a score of overall satisfaction. (See example in Figure 1.)

SECTION I: BACKGROUND

> **FIGURE 1**
>
> # Example: Rating Patient Satisfaction
> *Examples are selected and adapted from Press, 2002.[7] This is not a complete survey.*
>
> | **ADMISSION / ED / REGISTRATION** | very poor | poor | fair | good | very good |
> |---|---|---|---|---|---|
> | 1) Speed of admission. | 1 | 2 | 3 | 4 | 5 |
>
> **Your Room / the facility**
> 1. Noise level
> 2. Cleanliness
>
> **Your nurse**
> 1. Friendliness/courtesy
> 2. Skill
>
> **Your physician**
> 1. Friendliness/courtesy
> 2. Kept you informed
>
> **Discharge**
> 1. Instructions for care at home
>
> Other questions about your care: quality of communications, quality of information about medications, quality of pain control, effectiveness of staff coordination, etc.
>
> ## Algorithm (Example):
>
> - Overall satisfaction = average (average [admission], average [room], average [nurse], average [physician], average [discharge], average [other])
> - Or overall satisfaction = average (all questions)
> - Or overall satisfaction = average (each section, weighted by its presumed or empiric importance to patients)
> - Or other methodologies
>
> ---
> [7] op. cit.

Section I: Background

Option 2: Experience

Another approach is to evaluate specific, predefined aspects of the patient experience. Patients are asked whether certain events, deemed to be meaningful to most people on the basis of research, occurred consistently.

For example: "Did the discharge nurse explain how to take your medications at home?"; "Was the call light answered within five minutes?" Responses might be solicited in categories, such as "never," "seldom," "sometimes," "often," and "always." These data may be integrated into an overall "opportunity" score that essentially measures "defects" or missed opportunities to deliver the optimal experience of care. (See example in Figure 2.)

FIGURE 2 — **Example: Rating Patient Experience**

These examples and algorithms are adapted from the federal CAHPS survey,[8] and the new H-CAHPS survey, which is in pilot testing and is for research use only.

	never	sometimes	often	always
	1	2	3	4

Nurses
How often did nurses treat you with courtesy and respect?
How often did nurses explain things to you in a way you could understand?
How often did you get help (via the call button) as soon as you wanted it?

Doctors
How often did doctors spend enough time with you?

Environment
How often was room/bathroom kept clean?
How often was the area around your room quiet at night?

Experience
How often did you get help (bathing, using bathroom, etc.) as soon as you wanted?
How often did staff make sure that you had privacy?
How often did staff give you emotional support?
How often did staff work as a team?
How often did staff respond quickly with pain medicine?
How often did staff describe possible side effects of medicine?

Algorithm (Examples):

Overall satisfaction = average [average (environment), average (nurse), average (physician), average (experience), etc.]

---

[8] *Consumer Assessments of Health Plans Study (CAHPS®): Overview.* December 1998. Agency for Health Care Policy and Research, Rockville, MD. www.ahrq.gov/qual/cahps/

Option 3: Counting Complaints

Most hospitals have some method for receiving complaints or grievances, as required by the Medicare Conditions of Participation.[9] The JCAHO staffing effectiveness standard (see Section II, page 15) actually cites "complaints" as a suggested "clinical outcome" measure to be used for your staffing effectiveness analysis. As you will see below, there are advantages and disadvantages to this measure.

A possible measure of patient satisfaction could be a quantitative and/or thematic analysis of complaints and grievances if the hospital's data collection system is adequately sophisticated and if there are enough items submitted to generate a robust data set. The hospital would need to be sure that the data were collected systematically. In other words, you would need to be sure that all complaints and grievances were submitted to the database so that you have an accurate portrait of patterns and trends in patient perceptions.

In most hospitals, there is neither enough data (complaints) nor a sufficiently sophisticated classification and analysis system to ensure that "complaints" would be a meaningful measure of outcome.

Decision 2: How will you find out what your patients think? If the hospital uses convenience data, such as complaints or grievances, then you simply need to ensure that all patients know how to submit these concerns. In the vast majority of cases, however, this will not be an adequate approach to collect systematic, reliable, and valid data on patient perceptions. (This data can be a useful supplement to systematic survey data collection and can help further investigate potential problem areas and opportunities.)

The logistics of surveying can include mail, phone, or point-of-service surveys. Each has advantages and disadvantages. Mail surveys are relatively inexpensive, although costs can increase with multiple-wave surveys (e.g., sending a second or third survey to those who do not respond to the first mailing). Point-of-service surveys (paper and pencil, electronic kiosks, telephone touch-tone, or even patient video surveys similar to those used by hotels) are appropriate for brief encounters, such as outpatient visits, but literature suggests that they do not capture a thoughtful and complete response to a more extended interaction, such as a hospitalization. A short delay (a few days) before surveying is recommended for these encounters. Telephone surveys tend to yield fairly high response rates, but they're

---

[9] *www.cms.hhs.gov/manuals/pub07pdf/AP-a.pdf* Medicare Conditions of Participation Tag A752: *"The hospital must establish a process for prompt resolution of patient grievances and must inform each patient whom to contact to file a grievance."* Interpretive guidelines: § 482.13(a)(2)A *"patient grievance" is a formal, written, or verbal grievance that is filed by a patient when a patient issue cannot be resolved promptly by staff present.*

Section I: Background

biased, of course, toward patients who have a telephone. Due to the labor costs, they are likely to be more expensive than other modes.

All forms of patient surveys are biased toward consumers who communicate in the dominant language(s) in use at the provider site. It is important to consider whether surveying should be performed in more than one language. While not required by the current Office of Civil Rights (OCR), the OCR has criteria defining the size of a "limited English proficiency" population in the market for whom critical clinical documents (such as consent, discharge instructions, etc.) must be available in translation. These may be useful criteria for determining which populations need a survey in translation.[10]

The connection between patient satisfaction and staffing

No clear research results confirm a linear relationship between patient satisfaction and staffing. This is not a surprise, since patient satisfaction literature confirms that the key driver of satisfaction is not the quantity of patient interaction but the quality.[11]

Nonetheless, any hospital nursing manager or patient representative is likely to confirm that commonly articulated patient complaints include the following: "You don't have enough staff here," "The nurses are overworked," and "I can't find anyone to help me at shift change." And in fact, it is not unusual for staff to make the same observations, particularly after a day filled with additional admissions, a difficult patient/family interaction, or perhaps a systems failure of one sort or another. While this may seem an accurate anecdote to anyone working in the field, the challenge of staffing effectiveness is to develop a **systematic method** of assessing the adequacy of hospital staffing in meeting patients' needs.

Patterns of hospital staffing have moved cyclically over the past three decades. There has been a trend to use more assistive personnel under the supervision of nurses; in some settings, this has worked well, but in many it has been difficult to implement since nurses are not always trained or prepared to function as supervisors and may prefer a direct, hands-on patient care role. There has

---

[10] *www.hhs.gov/ocr/lep/ocrlepguidance.htm*
[11] Margaret Gerteis, Susan Edgman-Levitan, Jennifer Daley, & Thomas L. Delbanco (Editors). *Through the Patient's Eyes: Understanding and Promoting Patient-Centered Care* (Jossey-Bass, 1993).

SECTION I: BACKGROUND

also been a trend to develop different models for nursing care, varying from a dedicated nurse for a small group of patients, to a team approach in which a group of nurses rotates care of that group.

Simultaneously, since the implementation of Medicare Diagnosis Related Groups (DRGs) in 1983 and the subsequent aggressive care management strategies by most payers, lengths of stay have plunged and those who require inpatient care tend to be far more acutely ill than in the past. (Patients are admitted and discharged "sicker and quicker.")

Undeniable financial challenges, driven by reimbursement limits and increasing costs in areas such as medications, medical and surgical supplies, and energy resources, have led some hospitals to attempt to find lower-cost alternatives to registered nurses for some functions. In addition, the total supply of nurses has been stressed by fewer young people seeking nursing as a career, more professional options for trained nurses outside traditional acute care settings, and changes in lifestyle choices related to the overall increasing age of American nurses (presently in the mid-40s).

Several recent major national studies have confirmed a relationship between nurse staffing and selected clinical quality measures. Two of these studies have been published widely and have influenced legislation and accreditation efforts significantly. A 2001 federal Human Resources and Services Administration study provided a review of data from 1997 and concluded that "higher staffing levels for all types of nurses were associated with a decrease in adverse outcomes from 2% to 25%."[12] In 2002, two other studies published in major, peer-reviewed journals found similar results.[13,14]

Nationally, there has been enough concern about a nursing shortage and hospital staffing decisions that there have been state initiatives to legislate nurse-staffing ratios in nursing homes and hospitals. In California, for example, legislated staffing regulations effective in 2004 call for a ratio of 1 to 2 in critical care, ranging up to a ratio of 1 to 6 in medical/surgical (med/surg) units (falling to a ratio of 1 to 5 in 2005).[15]

---

[12] Press release dated April 20, 2001, at *www.hrsa.gov/newsroom* and full study at *www.bhpr.hrsa.gov/staffstudy.htm*

[13] Linda H. Aiken; Sean P. Clarke; Douglas M. Sloane; Julie Sochalski; Jeffrey H. Silber. "Hospital Nurse Staffing and Patient Mortality, Nurse Burnout, and Job Dissatisfaction." *Journal of the American Medical Association.* 2002;288:1987-1993.

[14] Jack Needleman, PhD; Peter Buerhaus, PhD, RN; Soeren Mattke, MD, MPH; Maureen Stewart, BA; and Katya Zelevinsky. Nurse-Staffing Levels and the Quality of Care in Hospitals. *New England Journal of Medicine,* vol. 346(22) May 30, 2002.

[15] *www.applications.dhs.ca.gov/regulations/store/Regulations/R-37-01%20reg%20text.doc*

Section I: Background

Certainly, patients and families are highly sensitive to perceived shortages of staff and tend to attribute many perceived care problems to inadequate staffing. There are other possible theories, however, that could account for patients' complaints about perceived problems with staffing. It is possible that staffing is adequate but communication is lacking: Staff are unable to inform patients effectively about what is being done for them. It is possible that nurse staffing is sufficient but that assistive personnel are in short supply, so nurses are not informed of patients' needs in a timely fashion. It is possible that patients' perceptions are accurate during a particular shift or on a particular unit, although staffing hospital-wide is adequate.

These trends, issues, and complexities are exactly what the new staffing effectiveness standards are intended to explore. Thoughtful attention to these standards can be instrumental to you in improving care at your hospital.

Why staffing effectiveness?

Many factors have led to concerns about whether there are enough clinical staff to deliver the outcomes our patients expect and desire. These factors include

- measurable shortages of nurses, pharmacists, radiology staff, and others

- sicker patients with shorter lengths of stay

- budget pressures in many health provider organizations

- increased consumerism and higher expectations

- more complex medical care, including invasive treatments and medication regimens, which demand more communication and patient education

- increasing research and evidence of a statistical association between at least nurse staffing and selected clinical outcomes

- increased staff workloads associated with documentation, training, and compliance efforts

In recognition of these and other concerns, the JCAHO developed an approach to assessing whether hospitals have enough staff to deliver desired outcomes. (The JCAHO is continuing to apply these

Section I: Background

principles to other settings besides hospitals. The staffing effectiveness standards for long-term care and assisted-living facilities go into effect in January 2004.)

Thus, among all the factors affecting accredited health care organizations like yours, one of the most significant was crafted by the JCAHO in 2002 when it established a standard requiring you to combine data on clinical screening indicators with HR screening indicators to assess staffing effectiveness. Helping you to meet JCAHO requirements and improve patient satisfaction is the focus of this book.

The relationship of patient satisfaction to staffing effectiveness

Many factors affect patient satisfaction. This book focuses specifically on the effect of staffing on patient satisfaction and how to use this relationship to improve care, as well as JCAHO assessment requirements. The JCAHO encourages organizational learning and supports the sharing of information to improve all aspects of patient care. Leaders should be able to implement improvements in the way care is designed and delivered, so that patients' needs and desires are met. This means that leaders have the freedom and resources to allocate time, energy, and money to priorities that patients have reported are important to them.

The public (your patients) is exposed to many forms of patient care quality information and is basing some of its health care decisions and choices on this information. It is urgent that health care leaders be aware of the perceptions of their patients and develop the capability to understand how to use data to take action.

The emergence of the staffing effectiveness standards

Staffing effectiveness is defined by the JCAHO as "the number, competency, and skill mix of staff as related to the provision of needed services." The standards were designed specifically to meet "the national need to address staffing issues at health care organizations" and to create "an objective and evidence-based approach to assessing the number, competency, and skill mix of their staff by linking staffing effectiveness to clinical outcomes."

JCAHO standards on staffing became effective July 1, 2002, for the acute care hospital setting. The primary purpose of the standards is to implement a process to study health care provider staffing and how it affects patient outcomes. The intent is to strengthen staffing effectiveness and improve patient outcomes in accredited organizations.

Section I: Background

A primary goal of the standards is to identify and ensure that a sufficient number of qualified staff are available to meet patient care needs. The standards do not require necessarily that organizations increase their data collection efforts or change actual staffing, but they do require that organizations analyze data to produce a factual analysis of the impact of staffing variation on patient outcomes. Many organizations already collect both HR and clinical data. Since July 1, 2002, it is expected, however, that organizations not only collect the data in discrete data sets but also use these measures in tandem to determine and adjust staffing plans.

The JCAHO's method for implementation is an approach that utilizes screening indicators that are sensitive to staffing effectiveness. Based on the consensus of a JCAHO expert panel and research group, the JCAHO lists 21 HR and clinical indicators for potential correlation.

You are not required to use the JCAHO measures exclusively. You must select two pairs of measures (each pair includes one HR and one clinical measure) and at least two of the four total measures (one of the HR measures and one of the clinical measures) from the JCAHO list. See below for more information on selection of measures. The single most important consideration in selecting measures is that they be driven by a meaningful and credible hypothesis that matters to your organization. The second most critical factor to consider is that the complexity and reliability of the data collection of the measures you selected are of greatest interest to your organization.

Caution
There is absolutely no element in the JCAHO's standards language or intent that would prescribe any specific staffing level. No one can ever say that your staffing does not "meet JCAHO standards" per se. Senior management, however, must be well aware of an important potential accreditation compliance concern related to staffing effectiveness: If your own analysis of the staffing effectiveness indicators, which you have carefully selected, leads you to the conclusion that your staffing is not optimal to achieve the targeted outcomes, then it is imperative that leaders respond to this finding.

JCAHO leadership standards require that the leaders provide a "sufficient number of qualified and competent persons to provide care." If your own analysis suggests that this is not occurring, obviously there must be a thoughtful and well-documented response. This could include staffing adjustments or further study to determine all the dynamics of the staffing/competence/outcome relationship, etc., but it cannot simply end with "continue to monitor." This issue is also discussed at the end of this book, with some suggestions for leaders regarding analysis, action, and associated documentation.

Section II
The Standards

Section II: The Standards

Description of the standards

All standards related to staffing effectiveness and data are integrated into the following chapters of the *Comprehensive Accreditation Manual for Hospitals (CAMH):* human resources, leadership, and performance improvement.

Although standard HR.2.1 is the "official" staffing effectiveness standard, organizations must also meet related standards in the leadership and performance improvement chapters, so you will want to pay close attention to these as well. For the purposes of this book, we refer to all of these standards as the "staffing effectiveness standards."

HR.2.1

The hospital uses data on clinical screening indicators in combination with human resource screening indicators to gauge or measure staffing effectiveness.

The intent of HR.2.1 states:
Hospitals examine multiple screening indicators relating to patient outcomes, including those for clinical and HR, to correlate staffing effectiveness.

1. Hospitals select a minimum of four screening indicators, two clinical and two HR. The focus is on the relationship between human resource and clinical/service indicators, with the understanding that no one indicator directly correlates with staffing effectiveness.

2. Hospitals select at least one of the HR and one of the clinical indicators from a list of Joint Commission–identified screening indicators. Hospitals identify additional screening indicators to understand the hospitals' own characteristics, specialties, and services.

Section II: The Standards

3. Hospitals determine the rationale for screening indicator selection. The measures should apply to the entire inpatient population; however, the JCAHO confirms that, as long as the four measures have been selected and implemented, it will not issue a recommendation if this goal cannot be met.

4. Hospitals include both direct and indirect caregivers in the HR screening indicators. Hospitals define which caregivers will participate in the HR screening indicators based upon what effect, if any, the absence of such caregivers is expected to have on patient outcomes.

5. Hospitals use the data collected and analyzed from the selected screening indicators to identify potential staffing effectiveness issues.

6. Hospitals establish a process for analyzing screening indicator data over time per measure (for example, the target ranges, trends over time, stability of process, external comparison data) and then in combination with other screening indicators, using methods such as matrix reports, spider diagrams, radar diagrams, and statistical correlations.

7. Hospitals analyze screening indicators at the level that's most effective for planning staffing needs, and they work with other areas in the hospital, if necessary. (By "level," the standards envision that some analysis will be performed with hospital-wide data, and other studies will be performed on a unit, population, or other basis. Later in this book, we will demonstrate how this can be done efficiently.)

8. The hospital reports at least annually to the leaders on the aggregation and analysis of data related to staffing effectiveness (PI.3.1.1) and any actions taken to improve staffing.

9. Hospitals demonstrate action taken, as appropriate, in response to analyzed data.

Your checklist for compliance with standard HR.2.1 then is to do the following:

- Develop your hypotheses regarding staffing and outcomes, with leaders of your organization.

- Select two different clinical and two different HR indicators that can be paired to test your hypotheses. Be sure that you include direct and indirect caregivers in your HR indicators.

- Provide rationale for indicator selection based on your patient population (document this in meeting minutes from your quality improvement [QI] committee, for example).

- Collect, analyze, and use data to identify potential staffing effectiveness issues. Be prepared to show the minutes of work teams and the QI committee, at whose meetings the data are presented and discussed. This process is exactly the same one that your organization uses for all other QI initiatives.

- Analyze indicators at the level (e.g., hospital-wide, population, unit, etc.) most effective for staff planning and in collaboration with other areas as applicable. This may be at departmental or team meetings.

- Provide annual summary report to leaders on aggregation and analysis of data (PI.3.1.1), as well as actions taken to improve staffing. The JCAHO has confirmed that this report can be integrated with your other annual reports on competence of staff and performance improvement, as well as other management and stewardship reports.

- Show evidence of action taken in response to analyzed data. This might include staff schedules, budgets, or continuing staffing effectiveness reports that display improvement.

Other related standards are PI.3.1, PI.3.1.1, PI.4.3, and LD.4.3:

PI.3.1

The organization collects data to monitor its performance.

- This is the core JCAHO standard requiring measurement and is not new. Remember that it does not require new measures; it is quite acceptable to use data already collected for other purposes and use it in new ways to meet the staffing effectiveness standards.

PI.3.1.1

The organization collects data to monitor the performance of processes that involve risks or may result in sentinel events.

- This standard requires that the hospital report to its leaders at least annually on the aggregation and analysis of data related to the effectiveness of staffing, and on any actions taken to improve staffing.

PI.4.3

Undesirable patterns or trends in performance and sentinel events are intensively analyzed.

- This standard has been revised to refer to staffing effectiveness. It ensures that staffing is considered as the hospital intensively evaluates undesirable patterns or trends in performance and sentinel events.

Section II: The Standards

LD.4.3

Leaders ensure that important processes and activities are measured, assessed, and improved systematically throughout the hospital.

- The intent of this standard has been revised to include priorities related to hospital-wide activities and staffing effectiveness, and relates back to HR.2.1 with respect to patient health outcomes.

Getting started

It is important to approach the creation of a process for data collection and analysis with some formality. The effort will take resources that should be well targeted, and the results of the analysis will be applied to one of the most important resource decisions of any hospital or health care provider: the deployment of staff. If you want to make effective change, you need to have reliable data and solid support for the strategy.

Staffing effectiveness should reflect concerns that are already incorporated into the strategic priorities of your organization: recruitment, retention, turnover, and patient clinical and satisfaction outcomes. What is more, the JCAHO explicitly expects that leaders be involved in the selection and use of these measures, so the process must include them.

Before you begin the process of selecting indicators and collecting data, discuss with your colleagues what needs and resources for data collection, analysis, and use already exist. HR leadership can identify what data are already being collected in that department. Consider overall issues that have been in the spotlight over the past year and may have affected patient satisfaction: Has there been a nursing shortage at your hospital? Have you used agency staff? Other data related to staffing are often easily obtained through the hospital's finance department (paid hours per day, variance in staffing compared to budget, etc.).

The second part of the equation is to evaluate your organization's strategies and issues related to patient satisfaction. In many cases, organizations have already established goals for improvement of patient satisfaction, perhaps for the entire organization or for key units or programs. You will want to build on any existing energy and focus that is dedicated to patient satisfaction.

It is advisable to direct this process under the oversight of your QI committee for several reasons. This committee constitutes the strategic leadership for quality measurement in your organization, so it will be key to the successful selection and use of measures. If you hope to effect organizational change on the basis of a relationship between staffing and patient satisfaction outcomes, you will need the committee's support. And while many state statutes encourage the collection of data to improve the quality of medical care while protecting the data from discovery, subpoena, or public disclosure, they require that the quality committee direct and manage the process. Check with experts in your own legal area to determine whether patient satisfaction and staffing data may be eligible for this privilege in your state.

Use the following checklist to guide your steps in this process.

Checklist for Meeting the Staffing Effectiveness Standards

1. Review and understand the JCAHO's staffing effectiveness standards.
2. Select the indicators for your patient population, including your entire inpatient population if possible. Use at least one clinical measure from the JCAHO's list and one HR measure from the JCAHO list. The others may be from the JCAHO's list or from your own list.
3. Define the indicators rigorously.
    - Determine site, department, and specialty ("level" of analysis).
    - Determine which direct and indirect caregivers to include. (Examples of direct caregivers include RNs, LPNs, nursing aides or assistants, respiratory and physical therapists. Indirect caregivers might include clinical support staff, such as infection control practitioners, staff educators, and staff in the dietary, maintenance, or housekeeping areas.)
4. Document rationale for indicator selection with appropriate leadership.
5. Determine sample range.
6. Collect data.
7. Plan analysis methods, including statistical process, control, and correlation.
8. Analyze and evaluate data—assess the correlation between/among indicators and opportunities for improvement.
9. Establish a staffing plan based on data.
10. Report to leadership.
11. Follow up and reevaluate staffing plan.

Section II: The Standards

A staffing effectiveness tool similar to the one in Figures 3 and 4 will assist you in coordinating the key steps in the process of collecting, analyzing, measuring, displaying, and using the information for staffing effectiveness.

The tool can be useful for reporting to your performance improvement (PI) committees, and it can assist you in ensuring that all areas of the necessary components are completed, tracked, recorded, and followed up on.

SECTION II: THE STANDARDS

FIGURE 3

Quality Improvement Planning and Monitoring Tool

Enter Hospital Name	
Quality Improvement Planning and Monitoring	Date:

PROCESS: Staffing Effectiveness

Overview, History, Why Important:
(Describe the pair of measures used to assess staffing effectiveness, why selected, hypothesis.)

Performance Dimensions and Goals:
(Describe the goal of the analysis: link these measures through correlation and other analyses to assess possible improvements in staff to improve outcome.)

Current Period Performance:
(Relevant data in graphic and/or tabular format [here or attached].)

Trend: Performance Over Time:
(Relevant data in graphic and/or tabular format [here or attached].)

FINDINGS AND CONCLUSIONS

Are the measures linked? What evidence of statistical relationship do you have?

Is staffing effective to achieve the desired outcome at this time? How do you know?

If not, what are team conclusions about potential areas for improvement?

What additional data, pilot studies, small-scale tests of change, etc. are needed?

STRATEGIES: Recommendations to be implemented/referred for action

Action *Including attention to new opportunities for improvement*	By Whom	By When

FOLLOW UP

Date:
Review data again
Update on referred recommendations
Report at unit/department meeting
Report to medical director/clinical leadership

Approved: _____

INCREASING PATIENT SATISFACTION WITH STATISTICAL CORRELATION

Section II: The Standards

FIGURE 4 — Staffing Effectiveness Data Plan Tool

HOSPITAL NAME

Quality Improvement Planning and Monitoring

STAFFING EFFECTIVENESS DATA PLAN

Name of measure set:

Inpatient care areas/patient populations *(describe population)*:

Types of practitioners/workers/providers *(describe practioners)*:

Indicator Pairs: *Enter indicator pairs (e.g., nursing hours and patient satisfaction)*

Staffing Effectiveness Measure Set 1 *(define hypothesis or area to explore)*:

1a. HR INDICATOR

Why important *(check one or more)*:	High Volume	High Risk	Problem Prone	Other Criteria
Selected from JCAHO list or hospital specific:	JCAHO list		Hospital-specific	
Caregivers *(check either or both)*:	Direct		Indirect	

Clearly define numerator or data element:

Clearly define denominator as relevant:

Sample: (define: 100% or sample):

Methodology (e.g., chart review, abstract from computerized reports):

Source (e.g., medical record, personnel system, surveys):

Benchmark, if any (source of external comparative data):

Frequency (monthly, quarterly, weekly, etc.)

1b. CLINICAL/SERVICE INDICATOR

Why important *(check one or more:)*	High Volume	High Risk	Problem Prone	Other Criteria

Clearly define denominator as relevant:

Sample: (define: 100% or sample):

Methodology (e.g., chart review, abstract from computerized reports):

Source (e.g., medical record, personnel system, surveys):

Benchmark, if any (source of external comparative data):

Frequency (monthly, quarterly, weekly, etc.)

SECTION II: THE STANDARDS

FIGURE 4 — Staffing Effectiveness Data Plan Tool (cont.)

2a. HR INDICATOR

Why important (check one or more:)	High Volume	High Risk	Problem Prone	Other Criteria

Selected from JCAHO list or hospital specific:	JCAHO list	Hospital-specific

Caregivers: direct, indirect (check either or both)	Direct	Indirect

Clearly define numerator or data element:

Clearly define denominator as relevant:

Sample: (define: 100% or sample):

Methodology (e.g., chart review, abstract from computerized reports):

Source (e.g., medical record, personnel system, surveys):

Benchmark, if any (source of external comparative data):

Frequency (monthly, quarterly, weekly, etc.)

2b. CLINICAL/SERVICE INDICATOR

Why important (check one or more:)	High Volume	High Risk	Problem Prone	Other Criteria

Clearly define denominator as relevant:

Sample: (define: 100% or sample):

Methodology (e.g., chart review, abstract from computerized reports):

Source (e.g., medical record, personnel system, surveys):

Benchmark, if any (source of external comparative data):

Frequency (monthly, quarterly, weekly, etc.)

Analysis plan (*describe briefly*):

Unit of measure (hospital wide, department, etc) (*describe briefly*):

Date Updated: _____

Approved By: _____

Section III

Step-by-Step Guide to Meeting the Staffing Effectiveness Standards

Section III: Step-by-Step Guide to Meeting the Staffing Effectiveness Standards

Choosing your indicators

So, now that you've been faced with the task of collecting data to meet the JCAHO's staffing effectiveness standards, your first question should be what data are you going to collect?

Each year, you must select two different **sets** of indicators to correlate: one HR indicator and one clinical indicator per set. The JCAHO's list of 21 staffing indicators (see Figure 5) provides a starting point for selecting your indicators. The JCAHO has, however, left considerable latitude to hospitals to refine the indicator definitions. (See glossary for possible indicator definitions.)

For example, the HR indicator "nursing hours" specifies neither the time period over which you are to count nursing care hours, nor the basis for measurement—e.g., "per patient day," "per acuity-adjusted patient day," etc. And it does not specify limiting the scope of the measures—that is, by unit or department rather than facility-wide. For practical reasons, unit- or department-based data will sometimes be more useful than more global groupings (e.g., facility-wide or an entire health care system). JCAHO expects, however, that the measures will encompass the entire inpatient population, if possible, and over time it is expected that this requirement will be enforced more rigorously.

FIGURE 5

JCAHO's 21 Clinical Service and HR Indicators

HR indicators

- Nursing care hours per patient day
- On-call or per-diem use
- Overtime
- Sick time
- Staff injuries on the job
- Staff satisfaction
- Staff turnover rate
- Staff vacancy rate
- Understaffing as compared to your staffing plan

Clinical service indicators

- Adverse drug events
- Family complaints
- Injuries to patients
- Length of stay
- Patient complaints
- Patient falls
- Pneumonias
- Postoperative infections
- Shock/cardiac arrests
- Skin breakdowns
- Upper gastrointestinal bleeding
- Urinary tract infections

Section III: Step-By-Step Guide to Meeting the Staffing Effectiveness Standards

Start by selecting the clinical indicator

Why should you start with the clinical indicator? The purpose of the staffing effectiveness standard is to improve patient outcomes. In general, it makes more sense for your quality committee to begin its deliberations by selecting outcomes that you wish to improve, and that you have reason to believe are possibly associated with staffing decisions.

Defining your clinical indicator: patient satisfaction

Important note: Although the JCAHO has provided a list of suggested indicators, you have the option of selecting a set of your own indicators for one of the two required correlations. This is particularly relevant if you are interested in examining patient satisfaction measures. Let's consider why.

"Patient complaints" may be a poor measure for staffing effectiveness analysis. As noted above, unless you have an extraordinarily systematic and comprehensive method of collecting patient complaints, your organization's data are likely to be sporadic and highly dependent on staff willingness to encourage staff to file a patient's complaint.

In order to assess staffing effectiveness, you will need data that are collected consistently and comprehensively. "Complaints" is probably not a measure that will meet these criteria in most organizations.

You probably already have goals established for patient satisfaction. Many, if not most, hospitals and providers have taken patient satisfaction measures quite seriously and have established strategic and/or tactical goals for performance levels and improvement. It is ideal to focus your staffing effectiveness effort on areas that are identified already as important areas to your organization.

Patient satisfaction data may be essentially "free." Since you already collect these data, there may be no additional cost to obtain them. There will be some additional effort involved in the analysis, of course, but this will be necessary for any staffing effectiveness assessment.

In considering which measure to use for patient satisfaction, you will want to keep these last two items in mind. Consider the following possible approaches, which would be applicable to most U.S. hospitals that collect systematic patient satisfaction data:

- Overall patient satisfaction (computed according to your instrument)

- Patient satisfaction with nursing

SECTION III: STEP-BY-STEP GUIDE TO MEETING THE STAFFING EFFECTIVENESS STANDARDS

- Patient satisfaction with other specific aspects or dimensions of care that you believe may be linked to staffing (education, emotional support, pain control, etc.)

- Patient satisfaction with tests and treatments

- Patient perceptions of delays in care

- Patients' reported "likelihood to return or recommend" your hospital, which is another measure of satisfaction

- Other measures that may be supported by your patient satisfaction instrument

With appropriate analysis and rationale, any of these could meet the JCAHO's definition of an acceptable clinical outcome measure. You will improve the likelihood that your process is useful, meaningful, and compliant if you ensure that you have engaged your management team in selecting measures that the organization genuinely wishes to improve, and considers valid and reliable.

Defining your hypotheses

At this point, as you finalize your selection of a patient satisfaction measure to use in your staffing effectiveness analysis, you should be developing a hypothesis that you plan to evaluate. This will help you decide how to measure patient satisfaction specifically, as well as which HR measure to select.

For example, review the following:

- "We think that patient satisfaction with nursing is probably related to the number of paid nursing hours per inpatient day."

    Implication: Clinical measure = an index of satisfaction with nursing
    HR measure = paid nursing hours per inpatient day
    *HR numerator: paid nursing hours**
    HR denominator: inpatient days

    *Be sure to specify whether you will include all full-time employees (FTEs) in the nursing department (including assistive staff, unit secretaries, and LPNs) or RNs exclusively.

- "We think that the percentage of very dissatisfied patients (regarding nursing care) is probably related to the percentage of agency and temporary staff in use at the time."

Section III: Step-By-Step Guide to Meeting the Staffing Effectiveness Standards

Implication: Clinical measure = percentage of patients rating "skill of nurses" as "very poor" or "poor"
Clinical numerator: number rating "skill of nurses" as "very poor" or "poor"
Clinical denominator: number responding to the question with any rating

or *Clinical measure = number of complaints about nursing*
Clinical numerator: raw number of complaints about nursing care per month
Clinical denominator: probably number of patient days (or patient discharges) per month—e.g., "number of opportunities to interact with nursing"

HR measure = percentage of agency and temporary staff
HR numerator: Paid agency/temporary hours this period (e.g., month)
HR denominator: Paid total staff hours this period

The following are other examples:

- "We think that overall satisfaction with the hospital is probably related to the number of total staffing hours in direct and indirect patient care departments that are filled by agency and temporary staff."
  Clinical measure = one of the satisfaction algorithms
  HR measure/numerator = agency/temporary staffing hour
  HR denominator = total staffing hours (include both direct and indirect staff, in selected departments)

- "We think that satisfaction with tests and treatments is probably related to the staff-hours-per-test-performed in the critical areas of radiology, cardiac services, and interventional programs."
  Clinical measure = satisfaction calculation related specifically to tests and treatments (depends on your patient survey tool)
  HR measure/numerator = staff hours (direct and selected indirect) in defined diagnostic and testing programs
  HR denominator = number of tests performed in those departments, probably monthly data

As is clear at this point, you now have an opportunity and responsibility to decide how to measure satisfaction.

SECTION III: STEP-BY-STEP GUIDE TO MEETING THE STAFFING EFFECTIVENESS STANDARDS

What Are Numerators and Denominators?

Why do we need to talk about numerators and denominators? Getting the right numerators and denominators when defining measures is critical to understanding the relationships you are going to investigate, specifically the relationships between HR and clinical indicators.

Specificity will strengthen your analysis, as in the following sample statement: We can count the number of patients discharged from orthopedics who rated nursing care as "poor" or "very poor" (numerator), and we can count the number of patients who responded to the survey in total (denominator). Thus, the measure of this particular indicator would be

$$\text{percent dissatisfied} = \frac{\text{number rating care "poor" or "very poor"}}{\text{number providing ratings in total}}$$

While some relationships among measures are obvious, easily defined, and straightforward to evaluate, others may not be.

So, what are numerators and denominators?
Numerators and denominators are used to describe three kinds of relationships: something (numerator) *divided by* something (denominator); something (numerator) per something (denominator); and the ratio of something (numerator) to something else (denominator).

When put in the form of a fraction, this might be a rate. For example, when looking at the number of patient complaints per month, the numerator is the complaints counted and the denominator is the number of months over which the complaints were counted.

If you are convinced that you can identify a representative *sample* from which to extrapolate your data, you can reduce the resources you will need to commit to collecting the data. For example, one

What Are Numerators and Denominators? (cont.)

could count the number of complaints on Unit 1 for a week and estimate monthly complaints by multiplying the count by the number of days in the month and dividing by seven (the number of days in a week or the period over which patient complaints were counted).

Bear in mind that the accuracy of the estimate will depend on the volume of events on a particular unit and the proportion you can afford to sample—smaller samples are generally less reliable than larger ones. In addition, the sample must be "representative."

For example, if you sample 10% of the medicine discharges for your hospital and produce a good-sized sample of 50 patients, but accidentally include only patients over age 65, you are unlikely to have a representative sample of patient satisfaction. (Older patients tend to be more satisfied than younger ones.)

Some rates are expressed as a percent. Simply stated, *percent* refers to something per 100 something else. Rates as percents are often used when the numerator is made up of cases also counted in the denominator, e.g., mortality, in which the numerator is persons who died and the denominator is the population of interest or at risk. For example, heart attack mortality among Minnesota men in 2002 (numerator) divided by the number of men who had heart attacks in Minnesota in 2002 (denominator). (See also the example of "percent dissatisfied patients" in the equation on the previous page.)

In our case study, we will examine patient satisfaction as a percentage score. Thus, we will sum the scores on all of the "nursing" questions for a single patient, then divide the total score by the number of questions on the survey in this section. This will work for any patient satisfaction survey, regardless of the number of nursing questions, as long as all of the questions have the same response scale and number equivalent (e.g., "very poor" (1) to "excellent" (6)). Then, we will compute an average overall patient satisfaction score for nursing by averaging this "index" score for all patients in the hospital in a given period of time, or all patients in an individual nursing unit or group of units in a period of time.

Some common approaches will include the following:
- An index of satisfaction as computed routinely on your survey tool. If this is already familiar to the staff in your organization and is already one of your goals, this is worth serious consideration.
  - Variations on this would include sub-indices, such as "index of satisfaction with nursing" or "index of satisfaction with personalized care," etc.
  - Another option is to select a single question from the survey that is of great importance to your organization and that you believe is related to staffing, and make this your exclusive focus. For example, "availability of the nurse" or "I received clear instructions on discharge as to how to take my medications."

- Percentage of patients rating care in the "top box" (best possible score) or "bottom box(es)" (lowest scores). (See page 37 for more about top box/botton box analysis.)
  - *Note:* In general, relatively few patients offer low ratings for patient satisfaction scores. If you want to focus on low scores, you may find that you will have better results by using more than one low-score category, such as "very poor" and "poor." Otherwise, you may have so few patients in the "low score" group that it is impossible to detect any relationship to staffing.

Now select the HR measure

Based on your outcome measure (some form of patient satisfaction measure) and your hypothesis of a relationship with staffing, you will have an idea as to which HR measure to select. You will repeat the same general selection process that you used to select your clinical measure:

- Determine what data are already collected in HR and/or finance (vacancy, turnover, paid hours for various staffing categories, agency utilization, number of patient admissions/days, etc.).

- Determine what the organization's improvement priorities are. If management is working hard on reducing turnover, then this is a measure on which you would be interested in focusing.

- Determine if your hypothesis can be evaluated with available data, or what will be required to manipulate or collect the additional data you may need.

It is important to determine which of all the possible measures has the greatest impact within your organization.

SECTION III: STEP-BY-STEP GUIDE TO MEETING THE STAFFING EFFECTIVENESS STANDARDS

Top Box/Bottom Box Analysis

Several strategies can be used to interpret satisfaction ratings:

- Responses for only the most satisfied (top category)
- Responses for the top two categories
- Responses for the bottom two categories
- Response for only the least satisfied (bottom category)

If the responses to satisfaction items look like the following table,

Item	Never	Rarely	Sometimes	Often	Always
Question 1	X				
Question 2	X				
Question 3				X	
Question 4					X
Question 5		X			
Question 6			X		
Question 7	X				
Question 8				X	
Question 9					X
Question 10			X		

- The interpretation for top box only will be the sum of "Always" items divided by the number of items. Q4 and Q9 are top box responses, so the satisfaction rate is 2 of 10 or 20 percent.

- Using the two top categories ("Often" and "Always"), we have 4 of 10 responses (Questions 3, 4, 8, and 9) or a satisfaction rate of 40 percent.

- Using the two bottom categories ("Never" and "Rarely"), we have 4 of 10 responses (Questions 1, 2, 5, and 7) or a dissatisfaction rate of 40 percent.

- Using the bottom box only (the "Never" choice), we have 3 of 10 responses (Questions 1, 2, and 7) or a dissatisfaction rate of 30 percent.

- Note that the center choice ("Sometimes") does not contribute to the satisfaction or dissatisfaction rates in the scheme presented above.

SECTION III: STEP-BY-STEP GUIDE TO MEETING THE STAFFING EFFECTIVENESS STANDARDS

Defining your HR indicator: nurse staffing

Some organizations have examined patient satisfaction and have concluded that it does not seem to bear a relationship to staffing measures. The literature on patient satisfaction suggests that one of the most critical intermediate variables driving inpatient satisfaction is the relationship with the bedside nurse. Thus, it may be most useful to focus on this relationship specifically.

If this is the hypothesis in your organization, you will wish to select a clinical measure that is specific to nursing. Similarly, you would want to choose a staffing (HR) measure that is related to the patient's access to the nurse. Initially, this could be nurse staffing (e.g, hours per patient day). A more sophisticated analysis could address the availability of support staff (unit secretary, nonlicensed assistive personnel, and even housekeeping staff), as they may have an effect on the ability of the nurse to meet the patient's needs at the bedside.

For this book's purposes, we've selected **inpatient satisfaction with nursing** (clinical indicator) and **nurse staffing** (HR indicator) as our two indicators for comparison. Using these indicators, we will illustrate how to collect, analyze, and evaluate data to demonstrate a correlation between staffing (nursing hours) and patient satisfaction. (Note that the JCAHO's requirements include references to indirect caregivers. If you decide to use *nursing hours* to correlate your patient satisfaction measure, you will want to make sure that your second pair of staffing effectiveness measures addresses indirect staff as well.)

Normalizing data

The JCAHO requires that your organization's analytical process be set up to review the screening indicator data per measure over time (such as patient days, hours, etc.). Of course, this is something you would want to do in any case. If you simply looked at raw staffing data, you might notice that there is a decline in staffing on certain days, such as weekends, when some volumes are lower. But this does not tell you anything about the degree to which patients have access to adequate available staffing, considering the census. By normalizing the data, you ensure that you are comparing "apples to apples," or consistent and fair staffing data, over time.

Thus, the goal of our example is to look at patient satisfaction, which is an average measured over all patients who responded to your survey, in relation to *"nursing hours per patient day."* Regardless of when the patient was discharged or treated, we will consider the nursing hours that were available to patients in the hospital on that day, considering the census. (For more information on time period and standardization, see Collecting and using your data, page 41.)

Section III: Step-By-Step Guide to Meeting the Staffing Effectiveness Standards

Although patient satisfaction with nursing, and nursing hours, are two reasonable indicators that may be selected by many hospitals, you should carefully examine your own facility to determine if these are appropriate for you. As noted above, it is important to choose measures that are meaningful to your organization. Whether you use our indicators or different indicators, this book and the companion spreadsheet will help you through the process of correlating whatever indicators you have chosen in order to meet JCAHO standards.

Outlining rationale

After you've defined your indicators, you will want to outline the rationale for the indicators you selected, as surveyors will almost certainly wish to discuss this. In order to document rationale, you may want to rank (by importance) your facility's concerns, using a priority scale. Priority can be determined based on data availability, volume, patient population, and strategic importance. You may have benchmark data suggesting that your organization could perform better on patient satisfaction, which has led you to identify this as a priority. The best possible driver for selection would be organizational goals established by senior management that indicate that your clinical outcome and HR measures are important strategically to your organization. It is quite acceptable, however, if the quality committee or another relevant group selects measures specific to the staffing effectiveness analysis.

As you choose your indicators for the clinical and HR areas, remember to look at the data you already have within your organization. Many times, the rationale for indicator selection will already be present in data you are collecting. For example, your HR department may already be tracking turnover rates and staff vacancy rates. On the other hand, an indicator should not be selected exclusively because your organization may already be collecting that data; it is essential to demonstrate the usefulness and relevance of the data.

Staffing and planning measures

As you select your indicators, the JCAHO requires you to keep a number of other factors in mind.

First, as noted previously, both direct and indirect caregivers must be included in your data collection for at least one of the two pairs of measures. As you prepare to collect data, you must define which caregivers should be included in your collection efforts based on the impact, if any, that the absence of such caregivers would have on patient outcomes.

In the current example, we have elected to focus exclusively on direct caregivers (nurses, LPNs, nurse aides, etc.). As a result, we would have to make sure that our second measure includes indirect caregivers. Alternatively, your hypothesis might be that the total staffing mix involved in patient care is instrumental in affecting patient satisfaction with the nurse, since it is the entire team that supports the nurse to deliver care. In that example, you would use a numerator measure that includes staff hours from nursing (including unit secretaries, unit-based transport staff, etc.), housekeeping, and perhaps even residents/interns.

The JCAHO also requires that the screening indicators be analyzed at the level most effective for planning staffing needs in the hospital and specifically to the patient population being served. The screening indicators will be implemented hospital-wide to see if there is a relationship in patient nursing satisfaction with overall staffing patterns.

The data can also be utilized on the nursing care units to demonstrate whether or not there is a correlation between staffing and satisfaction that may be different in different populations. (Most often, there will not be enough volume in an individual unit to conduct these studies locally on a monthly basis. You may wish to look at the data less often, perhaps quarterly. A more useful approach might be to consider grouping similar units for analysis—e.g., all medical units, surgical units, pediatric units, and obstetric units.)

In our example, this study is reserved for future "drill-down" after we conduct the high-level analysis. Such a "drill-down" can help to ensure that staffing plans will be based on identified issues relevant to that unit and in consideration of the patient population. Staffing needs may vary, depending on patient type. For example, geriatric medicine patients with multiple chronic illnesses may often have greater needs for discharge medication education and counseling from the nurse than acute care postsurgical patients. Your hypothesis might be that the geriatric patients could be less satisfied with nursing care, even if the staffing ratios are the same on both types of units.

Lastly, the JCAHO requires evidence that action is taken in response to analyzed data, as applicable. Your measures can include baseline target ranges, trends over time, stability of baseline data, and external comparison data, but measures must be reviewed in combination with the other screening indicators using statistical correlation methods. At the end of this book, we'll talk about possible actions you could take based on your analyzed data.

Completing the plan

The staffing effectiveness data plan will be your "map" to ensure compliance. You will complete the plan by clearly articulating the hypothesis and outlining your ideas for data collection and management.

Section III: Step-By-Step Guide to Meeting the Staffing Effectiveness Standards

Collecting and using your data

Before you actually begin the process of collecting data, however, you should first consider several questions:

- **What is the purpose of collecting your data, and what will your data be used for? Who will look at your data? What action will you take based on your data?**
  Before you even begin collecting data, you should decide your purpose. This will help you define what data to collect, and how to collect them.

  You'll probably have several reasons for collecting data. **Compliance with JCAHO standards,** as well as compliance with other regulatory organizations, such as CMS, may top your list of reasons. In that case, your purpose is compliance, and the data will be used as documentation for surveyors. You'll want to show that your data collection methodology was well thought out and based on your organization's specific concerns and areas of opportunity.

  You may also be collecting data to **advance your organization's PI efforts.** Your data will be used to measure your current processes and contribute to improving them when applicable. They should be reviewed by your QI/PI committees and will most likely result in some sort of presentation to leadership.

  Data can also be an important **staff training and behavior modification** tool. Collected data provide concrete examples of weaknesses and strengths. Showing staff members clear-cut data about the number of nosocomial infections spread from poor hand hygiene, for example, can be much more effective than just reminding them to wash their hands. Thus, you may want to consider collecting data that will help in staff training and, especially, in modifying behavior.

  From a patient satisfaction standpoint, you can't bring about change without first knowing the effectiveness of your current processes. Data collection—looking at your processes and collecting data about them—provides a critical source of measurement.

  For example, if you recently implemented a new patient communications program on a particular unit, you will want to have both pre- and post-program implementation data to examine the program's effectiveness (and to support why you implemented the program in the first place). If you can demonstrate the degree of improvement, you may be able to influence behavior rapidly.

Section III: Step-By-Step Guide to Meeting the Staffing Effectiveness Standards

The beauty of well-designed data collection is that you can (and you most likely will) have several purposes (and potential uses) for collecting data. If you set out with this in mind, you can usually collect data that will meet all of these goals (rather than having to set up several different data collection programs).

- **What data are available? What are your sources of data?**

    Before you begin collecting any data, you should first find out what data already exist and who has them. You'll probably find that your hospital has many data sources. Chances are, if you're an accredited hospital, you're already collecting data to meet the JCAHO's PI requirements and to meet your own organizational PI initiatives.

    Quality leaders and data analysts within your hospital would be obvious people to ask for existing data. Other sources of data include patient records; patient and staff satisfaction surveys; department logs and shift reports; HR, nursing, and finance departments; and infection control case management and risk management information.

    With the indicators used in our case study, very little unique data collection should be needed in most organizations. Staffing data, patient days, and patient satisfaction data are all usually routinely available from existing systems, and your task will be to simply abstract the data from the official source systems and build the relationships.

- **For what time period should you collect data? How many data points should you consider?**

    One of the first things you will want to consider as you begin to collect data is what time period should be examined. Although the JCAHO's staffing effectiveness standards do not mention time period specifically, it is likely that surveyors will look for evidence in your rationale for why you chose to collect the data over a specific time period.

    Your time period for data collection will depend, in part, on the clinical indicator you plan to use in examining any correlation of staffing to patient outcomes. Collecting data over shorter periods of time is possible for more frequently observable patient outcomes.

    For example, if one were to monitor wait times in a busy emergency room, there would be a sufficient number of events within days to support your analysis. Patient satisfaction data should be fairly plentiful within a short time if your survey methodology has a reasonably high response rate. In most cases, monthly analysis of patient satisfaction data should be feasible for a hospital-wide aggregation.

Section III: Step-by-Step Guide to Meeting the Staffing Effectiveness Standards

If you want to analyze staffing effectiveness for individual units or departments within the hospital, however, it is much less likely that there will be a sufficient number of surveys in a given month. These areas may be analyzed more reliably on a quarterly basis.

As you look at one unit or the whole organization over a period of time, you'll have a measurement for the time period you select, and that measurement constitutes a data point. The duration of the time period can be days, weeks, months, or years. In an ideal statistical world, you would have at least 30 responses in each data point. These would then strengthen your ability to draw conclusions on the monthly data points over the duration of your study.

Thus, if you are looking at daily data on one unit over a month's time, you'll have about 30 "responses" for the month's "data point" (depending on the number of days in the month), each based on patient satisfaction survey responses for patients discharged from that unit. If you opt to look at several units as a cluster (for instance, medical units, surgical units, obstetrics (OB), etc.), you'll have a measurement for each cluster.

The strategy for evaluating performance outlined in the JCAHO's PI standards is to begin by gathering data. When you have 24 data points (e.g., two years of monthly data), you will typically add new data points and at the same time drop the oldest data points. This keeps the trend analysis more manageable and relevant.

Perhaps you do not have two years of historical data on the measures of interest. Not having historical data does not preclude your studying the staffing/patient outcomes relationships. You need to start somewhere. If you have only six months' worth of data (that's monthly data—so that would mean you have only six data points), you can still collect the data and begin to analyze it. **You should be very cautious, however, when taking action based on a small number of measurements.**

If your small sample size yields noteworthy results—suggesting, for instance, that there is a relationship between patient satisfaction data and your staffing measure—then you will need to decide if action is appropriate based on the limited data you have available.

Depending on the strength of the results and the significance of your organization's concerns related to patient satisfaction, it might be best to go back and collect more data that corroborate your findings before taking any action. Or, if the situation is particularly alarming, it may be best to make an immediate change and continue to collect and analyze data.

From a perspective of leadership responsibility (as well as JCAHO compliance), this decision can be made only by senior leaders on the basis of available information and statistical insight.

You should also keep in mind that time period affects each of the JCAHO HR and clinical indicators—even those that appear to involve only a single measurement, such as number of dissatisfied patients, or average satisfaction level, etc. All these indicators have an implied period of time over which the events occur. For example, the indicator "patient satisfaction" actually refers to the average satisfaction level for a given time period (week, month, quarter).

For the purposes of comparing two indicators, your indicators should be based on the same period of time—this is called "standardizing." In our case, we're looking at patient satisfaction averaged over a month, and nursing hours per patient day, also computed on the basis of the same month.

Why must you look at nursing hours per patient day rather than just nursing hours? Nursing hours and nursing hours per patient day are two different measures. Just because you have the same number of nurses on a unit on Day 1 and Day 2 does not mean that you have the same number of nursing hours available for any given number of patients, since you may not have the same number of patients on those two days. This difference may or may not affect your patient satisfaction levels; the purpose of our "staffing effectiveness" analysis is, in fact, to assess this possibility.

For example, let's look at Unit 3 in Hospital ABC. Unit 3 drops from a near-capacity 20 patients on Day 1 to 15 patients on Day 2. The number of nursing hours on the unit remains the same on both days—11 full-time nurses across three shifts. While the number of nursing hours is the same for both days, the demand for patient care was greater on Day 1. In fact, the nursing hours per patient day on Day 1 were 88/20 (11 full-time nurses x 8-hour day divided by 20 patients) = 4.4 nursing hours per patient day. On Day 2, however, the nursing hours per day were 88/15 (11 full-time nurses x 8-hour day divided by 15 patients) = 5.9 nursing hours per patient day.

The HR indicator "nursing hours per patient day" describes the resources applied to the resource demand within a prescribed period of time. Resource allocation across patient care units has now been defined and can be compared. This will be important in assessing the relationship of nursing hours to patient satisfaction—that is, whether differences in resource allocation (nursing hours per patient day) have an impact on patient satisfaction.

SECTION III: STEP-BY-STEP GUIDE TO MEETING THE STAFFING EFFECTIVENESS STANDARDS

- **What will be your sample size? What is your data range for collection?**

    Your sample size and data range will be based on your answers to the questions about purpose. If your goal is to use the data for staff training purposes, you may want to collect data specific to the unit/units where you are training. If your goal, however, is overall patient satisfaction for the hospital, you may want to look at data on a facility-wide level (to get a sense of correlation of the indicators and results to patient satisfaction), as well as unit-by-unit (for future comparison and use at the unit level).

    If you opt to use a clinical indicator where there may be infrequent observable patient outcomes (such as shock or cardiac arrest), an alternative data collection strategy might be to group similar patient care units together for analysis so that there is a sufficient volume of events over which to measure differences in frequency of outcomes relative to differences in staffing parameters. If three med/surg units have very similar types of patients, it may be appropriate to combine the units for analysis of the clinical indicator and your HR indicator. **This is unlikely to be an issue if patient satisfaction is your clinical outcome measure.**

    In our case, an area that can be challenging is the intensive care unit (ICU). Most patient satisfaction surveys are administered after discharge, and patients are asked to reflect on the unit from which they were discharged. As a result, ICUs receive few, if any, survey results. They may need to be excluded from analysis, or you may wish to explore a customized survey approach for these areas, or perhaps to consolidate them into one group for analysis of the few surveys that they do receive.

    If you opt to use a clinical indicator where there are frequent observable patient outcomes (such as satisfaction survey results, or medication errors), you may want to devise a sampling methodology (See box on next page). As noted above, however, patient satisfaction data are usually already collected and readily available, so you will be able to use 100% of the surveys that are returned.

What Is Sampling?

When you are counting many events, when they are occurring frequently (perhaps medication errors or patient satisfaction survey scores), and if there is a cost for data collection, you may want to devise a sampling methodology. You will need to apply your methodology uniformly to guarantee statistically sound results.

If your patient satisfaction data are expensive to collect, or are collected manually, you may not wish to survey every patient.

For example, in one month, you might collect survey results and nursing hours per patient day on every date that is a multiple of three (the 3rd, 6th, 9th, 12th, etc., yielding 10 data points per month). On second shift, you record nursing hours per patient day and survey results on every date that is one less than a multiple of three (the 2nd, 5th, 8th, 11th, etc., also yielding 10 data points per month, depending on the month). Finally, on third shift, you record survey results and nursing hours per patient day on every date that is one more than a multiple of three (the 1st, 4th, 7th, 10th, etc., yielding 10 or 11 data points per month). You have thus created a random, uniform methodology for sampling HR and clinical activity on a patient care unit for one month that generates about 30 data points instead of one.

If events occur less frequently than once a day, you may need to consider alternative strategies for collecting your data— that is, for longer periods of time or across all shifts, for example.

SECTION III: STEP-BY-STEP GUIDE TO MEETING THE STAFFING EFFECTIVENESS STANDARDS

Our data

For the purpose of this book, we've already determined the purpose and use of our two indicators. We will be discussing the process of collecting and analyzing sample data from a hypothetical hospital, using the following guidelines:

- We have selected two indicators—patient satisfaction with nursing care and nursing hours—to look at the relationship between the indicators, staffing effectiveness, and the relationship to patient-perceived outcomes.

- We will be collecting data for three reasons: to look for a possible relationship between patient satisfaction and nursing hours; to meet the JCAHO standard; and to evaluate if there is a correlation between the clinical indicator (inpatient satisfaction, in this example) and staffing effectiveness. Ultimately, we will be collecting data to implement actions to improve patient satisfaction, if in fact there is a relationship between our two indicators.

- We've collected and calculated a month's worth of daily data for 10 patient care units with 20 beds each over 18 months. Patient satisfaction data comes from surveys, and nursing hours data are available through financial data produced by the organization's routine reporting systems (paid hours by job class, and number of patient days according to the census).

- For comparability, we've looked at each indicator over a common period of time. Thus, our derived indicators are nursing hours per patient day, computed over a month, and patient satisfaction for the same month. Patient day data may be available through your finance or health information management departments.

- We will be looking at all patient satisfaction results each month (rather than a sample).

- We will be collecting data only in relevant med/surg units. In our example, we have excluded data from the ICU because this could skew our data. ICUs tend to receive few patient surveys since few patients are discharged directly from ICUs, and survey results are unlikely to be representative.

Recording your data

You can organize your data using a number of different tools. You will, however, certainly want to organize your data in a table that can be stored electronically. We've chosen to do this in an Excel spreadsheet because it will allow us to calculate statistical functions, such as mean, median, mode, and standard deviation automatically (once we have entered the appropriate formulas), as well as create graphs for presentation. This book's companion spreadsheet already contains formulas and is customizable for most facilities, so you can add your own headings, units, etc. (The formulas, however, are write-protected and will not change.)

Note: **In order to enter data, you should save the Excel file from the CD in the back of this book to your hard drive or network storage area. The basic spreadsheet looks like the sheet illustrated in the following screen shots (not including the data).**

Regardless of the tool you use, yours should include several standard sections. Before entering any of the data you have collected, you should create column headings that accurately describe the data you plan to enter. Screen Shot 1 shows the sample spreadsheet we will be using to record our data on patient satisfaction and nursing hours. Let's use our sample spreadsheet to walk through the columns and rows one by one.

Section III: Step-By-Step Guide to Meeting the Staffing Effectiveness Standards

Setting up your spreadsheet

Spreadsheet headings (rows 1 and 2)

If you are using the book's companion spreadsheet, spreadsheet headings should already be entered in rows 1 and 2. Note that the first row (row 1) contains column headings that are generic descriptions for the columns, and the second row (row 2) contains column headings specific to the data entered in the spreadsheet. Most likely, your row of generic descriptions will be the same as those listed in row 1 of our spreadsheet, regardless of the indicators you choose. The headings in row 2, however, are specific to the indicators you select. Our spreadsheet's headings are pre-entered based on patient satisfaction and nursing hours. You must change these headings if you have selected a different set of indicators.

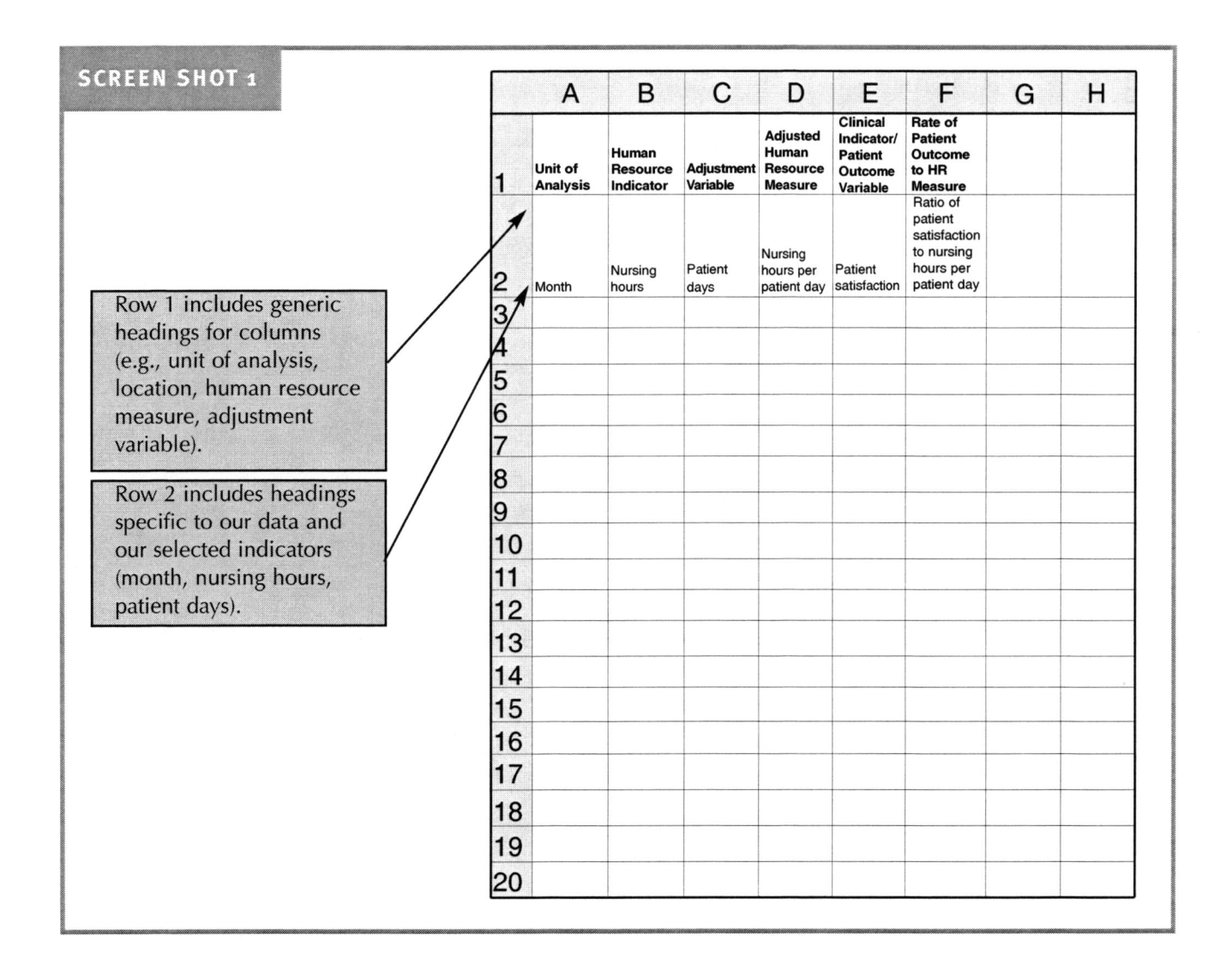

SCREEN SHOT 1

	A	B	C	D	E	F	G	H
1	Unit of Analysis	Human Resource Indicator	Adjustment Variable	Adjusted Human Resource Measure	Clinical Indicator/ Patient Outcome Variable	Rate of Patient Outcome to HR Measure		
2	Month	Nursing hours	Patient days	Nursing hours per patient day	Patient satisfaction	Ratio of patient satisfaction to nursing hours per patient day		
3								
4								
5								
6								
7								
8								
9								
10								
11								
12								
13								
14								
15								
16								
17								
18								
19								
20								

Row 1 includes generic headings for columns (e.g., unit of analysis, location, human resource measure, adjustment variable).

Row 2 includes headings specific to our data and our selected indicators (month, nursing hours, patient days).

SECTION III: STEP-BY-STEP GUIDE TO MEETING THE STAFFING EFFECTIVENESS STANDARDS

Column A

You will first need a column to identify your unit of analysis (e.g., time period, patient care unit, specialty, etc.) for which you intend to analyze the relationship between HR and clinical indicators. In our case, the unit of analysis is a time period (one month), identified in column A of Screen Shot 2.

If you choose to work with only one time period and record HR and clinical indicator data across locations, you will want to designate the first column as a location (patient care unit, for example) rather than a time period. The location may be clusters of similar patient care units, or clinical departments, or whatever standard grouping you choose. Gathering HR and clinical indicator data across locations will enable you to compare performance on these measures. Our instructions, however, should still apply to the data you enter in your columns.

SCREEN SHOT 2

Column A identifies unit of analysis (in our case, month).

	A	B	C	D	E	F	G	H
1	Unit of Analysis	Human Resource Indicator	Adjustment Variable	Adjusted Human Resource Measure	Clinical Indicator/ Patient Outcome Variable	Rate of Patient Outcome to HR Measure		
2	Month	Nursing hours	Patient days	Nursing hours per patient day	Patient satisfaction	Ratio of patient satisfaction to nursing hours per patient day		
3								
4								
5								
6								
7								
8								
9								
10								
11								
12								
13								
14								
15								
16								
17								
18								
19								
20								

Section III: Step-By-Step Guide to Meeting the Staffing Effectiveness Standards

Column B and column C

You will need at least one column to track the values of your HR indicator over the period of time that you have selected. Column B in our spreadsheet will be used to track the value of our HR indicator, nursing hours. In the case of nursing hours, remember that you are actually looking at nursing hours per patient day. Nursing hours and patient days must be counted each month to generate this number. Thus, column C in Screen Shot 3 will be used for recording patient days. (In this case, the denominator is also known as the adjustment variable.)

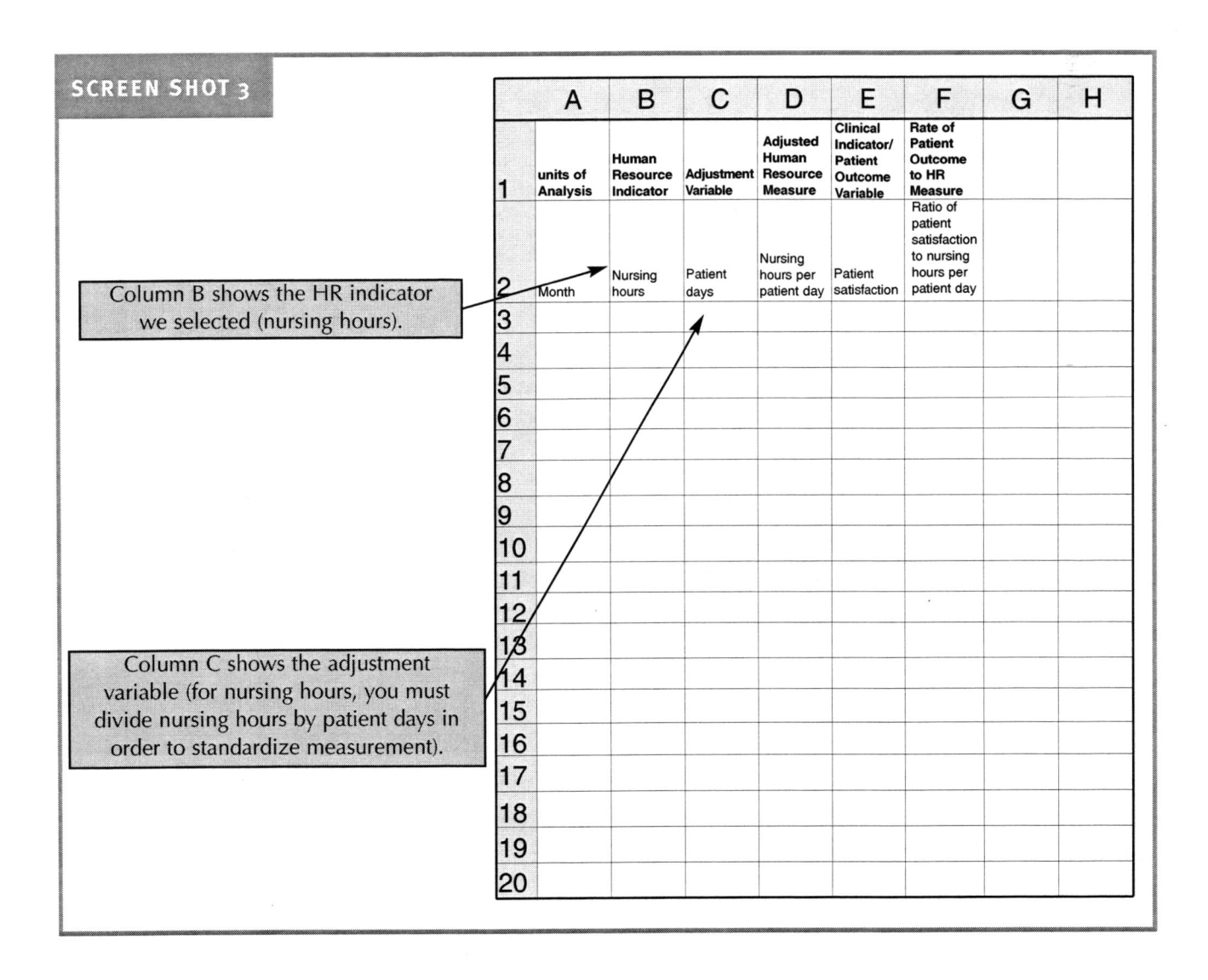

SCREEN SHOT 3

	A	B	C	D	E	F	G	H
1	units of Analysis	Human Resource Indicator	Adjustment Variable	Adjusted Human Resource Measure	Clinical Indicator/ Patient Outcome Variable	Rate of Patient Outcome to HR Measure		
2	Month	Nursing hours	Patient days	Nursing hours per patient day	Patient satisfaction	Ratio of patient satisfaction to nursing hours per patient day		
3								
4								
5								
6								
7								
8								
9								
10								
11								
12								
13								
14								
15								
16								
17								
18								
19								
20								

Column B shows the HR indicator we selected (nursing hours).

Column C shows the adjustment variable (for nursing hours, you must divide nursing hours by patient days in order to standardize measurement).

Section III: Step-By-Step Guide to Meeting the Staffing Effectiveness Standards

Column D

Column D is used for calculating the ratio of nursing hours to patient days (nursing hours per patient day). If you are using our spreadsheet, column D already contains the formula for calculating nursing hours per patient day (the adjusted HR measure). See Screen Shot 4.

This formula is simple: The HR measure divided by the adjustment variable = the adjusted HR measure; or, using our indicators, nursing hours (column B) divided by patient days (column C) = nursing hours per patient day (column D). If you choose to use an HR indicator other than nursing hours, you will need to label column D differently—or you may not need this column at all.

SCREEN SHOT 4

	A	B	C	D	E	F	G	H
1	Units of Analysis	Human Resource Indicator	Adjustment Variable	Adjusted Human Resource Measure	Clinical Indicator/ Patient Outcome Variable	Rate of Patient Outcome to HR Measure		
2	Month	Nursing hours	Patient days	Nursing hours per patient day	Patient satisfaction	Ratio of patient satisfaction to nursing hours per patient day		
3								
4								
5								
6								
7								
8								
9								
10								
11								
12								
13								
14								
15								
16								
17								
18								
19								
20								

Column D shows the adjusted HR measure (nursing hours per patient day) once you have standardized.

Column E

You will need at least one column to track the values of your clinical indicator, whose relationship to the HR indicator you are analyzing. In our case, the clinical indicator is patient satisfaction. We are standardizing measures (meaning we are looking at nursing hours per patient day calculated over a month, and patient satisfaction averaged over the same month), but patient satisfaction data are already calculated for us each month by our survey analysis process (as is the case in virtually all hospitals and patient satisfaction analysis systems). Thus, we don't have to perform any additional calculations and can place the patient satisfaction measure in column E, as shown in Screen Shot 5.

SCREEN SHOT 5

	A	B	C	D	E	F	G	H
1	Unit of Analysis	Human Resource Indicator	Adjustment Variable	Adjusted Human Resource Measure	Clinical Indicator/ Patient Outcome Variable	Rate of Patient Outcome to HR Measure		
2	Month	Nursing hours	Patient days	Nursing hours per patient day	Patient satisfaction	Ratio of patient satisfaction to nursing hours per patient day		
3								
4								
5								
6								
7								
8								
9								
10								
11								
12								
13								
14								
15								
16								
17								
18								
19								
20								

Column E tracks the values of our clinical indicator, which, in our example, is patient satisfaction.

If you selected a measure that does require standardization, you will use a different approach. For example, if you choose "number of dissatisfied patients per patient day," you will again need three columns in order to derive the adjusted patient outcome measure (in our case, patient dissatisfaction ratings per 1,000 days).

SECTION III: STEP-BY-STEP GUIDE TO MEETING THE STAFFING EFFECTIVENESS STANDARDS

Using our existing spreadsheet, these columns would be column E, column F, and column G. Column E would contain the number of patients with a "dissatisfied" rating (the clinical indicator), column F would contain the number of patient days (the denominator/adjustment variable), and column G would calculate the ratio of patient dissatisfaction to patient days (patient dissatisfied ratings per 1,000 patient days). **Because we do not need to standardize our clinical measure, however, we will be using column F for a different purpose.**

Column F

Column F, the ratio of patient satisfaction to nursing hours per patient day, is the final column in the spreadsheet. If you're using our spreadsheet, it should fill in the results automatically after you've entered data in columns B, C, and E. The formula for this calculation is to divide your clinical indicator (in our case, patient satisfaction/column E) by your HR indicator (in our case, nursing hours per patient day/column D) and multiply by a scaling factor of 100. In our case, we need to use 100 as a scaling factor to have a number that is greater than one. Without scaling, the number would be 0.1886; however, per 100 nursing hours, the number would be 18.86. This is simply for ease of use. The mathematical relationships are unchanged, but integers are easier for us to work with.

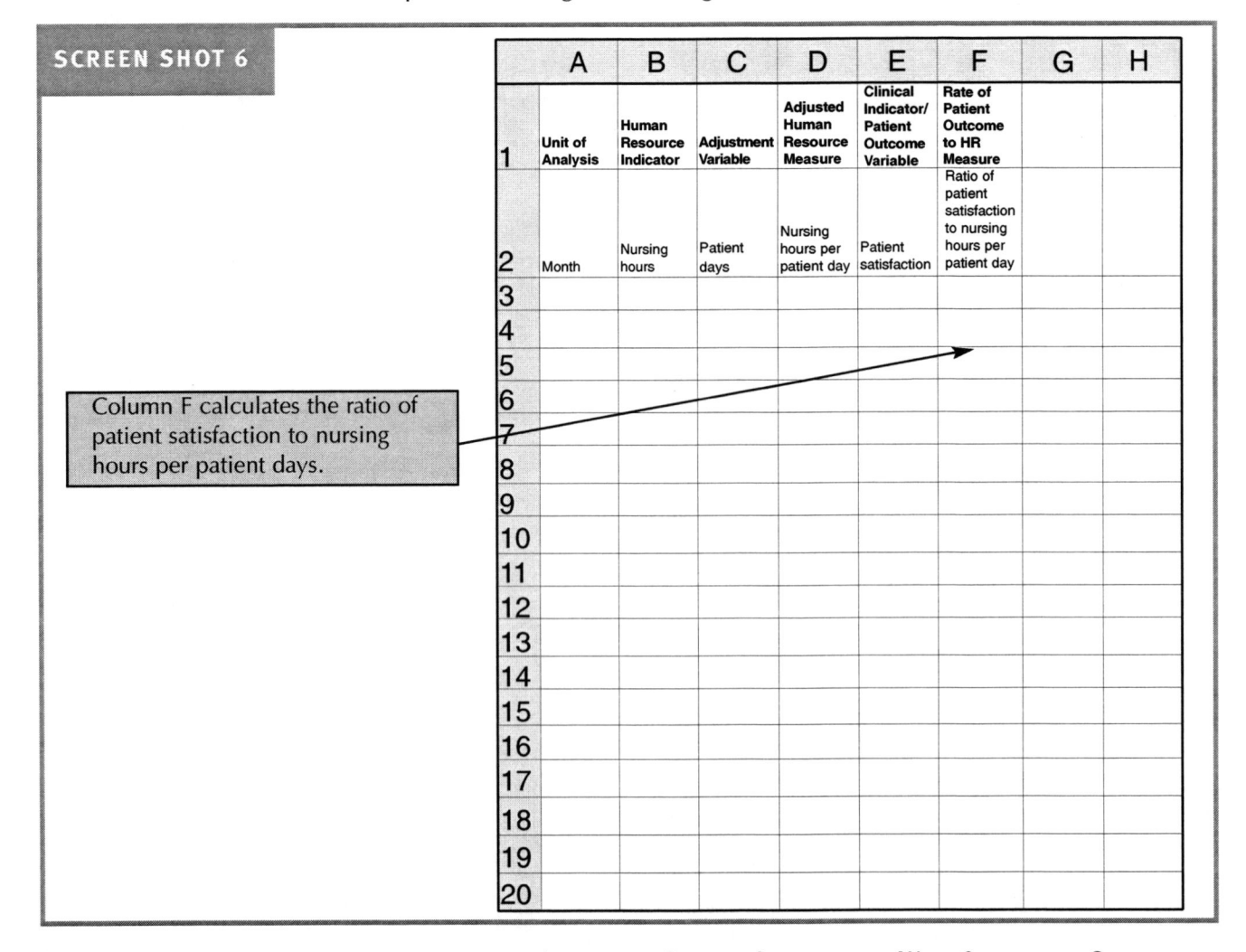

SCREEN SHOT 6

Column F calculates the ratio of patient satisfaction to nursing hours per patient days.

	A	B	C	D	E	F	G	H
1	Unit of Analysis	Human Resource Indicator	Adjustment Variable	Adjusted Human Resource Measure	Clinical Indicator/ Patient Outcome Variable	Rate of Patient Outcome to HR Measure		
2	Month	Nursing hours	Patient days	Nursing hours per patient day	Patient satisfaction	Ratio of patient satisfaction to nursing hours per patient day		
3								
4								
5								
6								
7								
8								
9								
10								
11								
12								
13								
14								
15								
16								
17								
18								
19								
20								

Section III: Step-By-Step Guide to Meeting the Staffing Effectiveness Standards

Why are the results in column F relevant? We are looking at the relationship between our clinical measure (patient satisfaction for a given month) as the numerator of the ratio and our HR measure (nursing hours per patient day) as the denominator of the ratio (column F).

If this relationship is uniform across patient care units, or does not change over time, then we would conclude that nursing hours do appear to have an effect on patient satisfaction—that is, increases in nursing hours yield associated increases in patient satisfaction resulting in a ratio that does not change.

Entering your data

Once you have set up the spreadsheet that you will be using to record your data, you are ready to begin entering data. For the purposes of showing you how to enter data, we will be populating our companion spreadsheet with hypothetical sample data based on our two indicators: patient satisfaction (clinical indicator) and nursing hours per patient day (HR indicator).

Again, let's go through our spreadsheet column by column. Look at Screen Shot 7.

SECTION III: STEP-BY-STEP GUIDE TO MEETING THE STAFFING EFFECTIVENESS STANDARDS

Column A

Column A represents time. You could represent your time periods as Month 1, Month 2, Month 3; or Jan '03, Feb '03, etc.

If you are collecting data from a number of locations, as we are here, you just need to enter the names of those locations in the companion spreadsheet. If you have opted to look at each of many units over a single period of time, you will need to enter location labels in the "Unit of Analysis" column. For example, you might use units 1-10; or Med/Surg 3E, Med/Surg 3N, Cardiac Care 2S, and so on.

SCREEN SHOT 7

	A	B	C	D	E	F	G	H
1	Units of Analysis	Human Resource Variable	Adjustment Variable	Adjusted Human Resource Measure	Patient Outcome Variable	Rate of Patient Outcome to HR Measure		
2	Month	Nursing hours	Patient days	Nursing hours per patient day	Patient satisfaction	Ratio of patient satisfaction to nursing hours per patient day		
3	Jan.01							
4	Feb.01							
5	Mar.01							
6	Apr.01							
7	May.01							
8	Jun.01							
9	Jul.01							
10	Aug.01							
11	Sep.01							
12	Oct.01							
13	Nov.01							
14	Dec.01							
15	Jan.02							
16	Feb.02							
17	Mar.02							
18	Apr.02							
19	May.02							
20	Jun.02							

Column A illustrates the entering of time or month.

Section III: Step-by-Step Guide to Meeting the Staffing Effectiveness Standards

Column B and column C

Once you have entered your "Unit of Analysis" in column A, you will need to enter HR and clinical data into subsequent columns. (See Screen Shot 8.) Remember that for our indicators, we are standardizing nursing hours by using the denominator patient days. Thus, our spreadsheet needs three columns to determine the adjusted HR indicator. Those columns are monthly nursing hours (column B), total patient days for the same one-month period (column C), and nursing hours per patient day (column D). You will enter data in the first two columns, and column D will be automatically calculated.

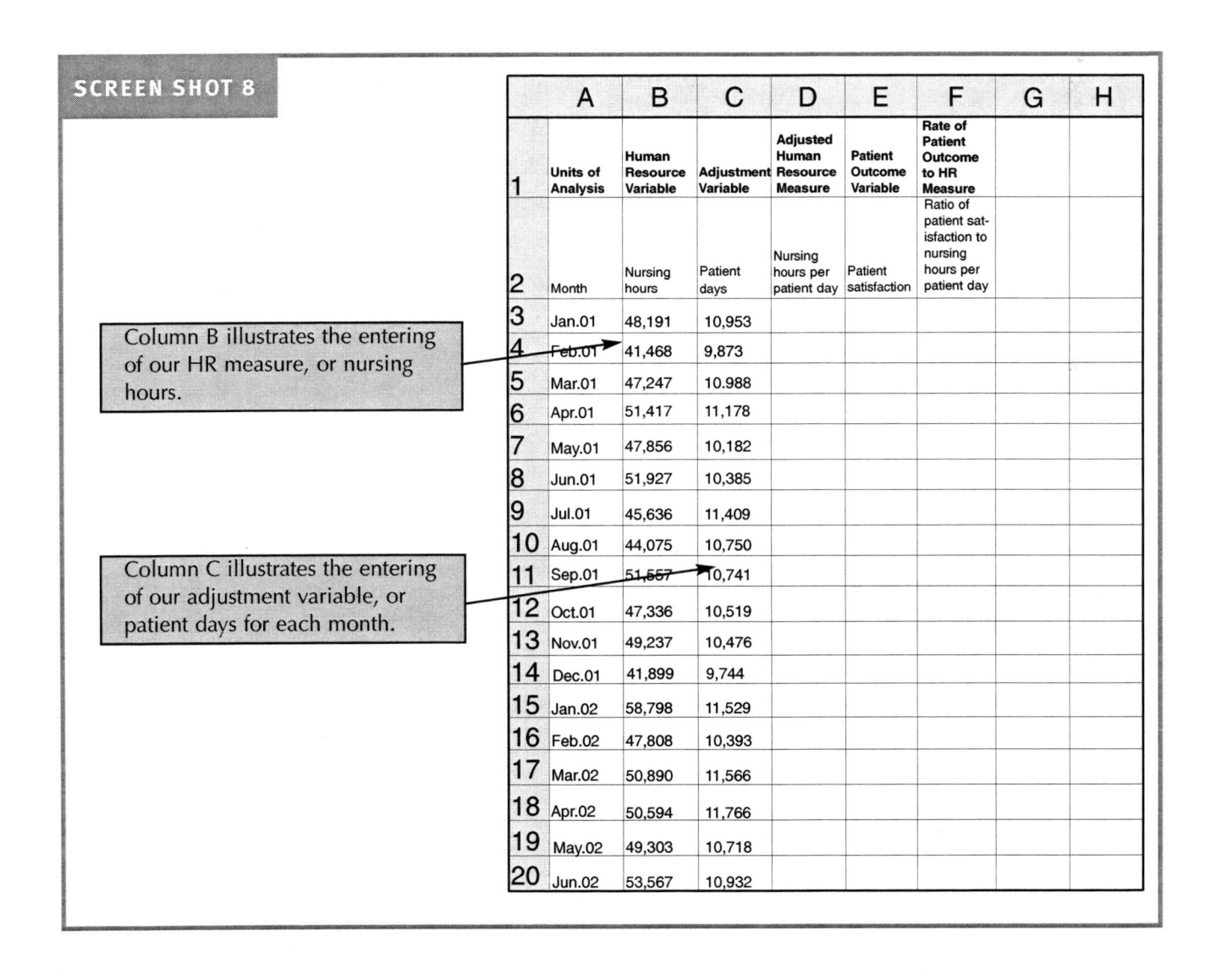

SCREEN SHOT 8

	A	B	C	D	E	F	G	H
1	Units of Analysis	Human Resource Variable	Adjustment Variable	Adjusted Human Resource Measure	Patient Outcome Variable	Rate of Patient Outcome to HR Measure		
2	Month	Nursing hours	Patient days	Nursing hours per patient day	Patient satisfaction	Ratio of patient satisfaction to nursing hours per patient day		
3	Jan.01	48,191	10,953					
4	Feb.01	41,468	9,873					
5	Mar.01	47,247	10.988					
6	Apr.01	51,417	11,178					
7	May.01	47,856	10,182					
8	Jun.01	51,927	10,385					
9	Jul.01	45,636	11,409					
10	Aug.01	44,075	10,750					
11	Sep.01	51,557	10,741					
12	Oct.01	47,336	10,519					
13	Nov.01	49,237	10,476					
14	Dec.01	41,899	9,744					
15	Jan.02	58,798	11,529					
16	Feb.02	47,808	10,393					
17	Mar.02	50,890	11,566					
18	Apr.02	50,594	11,766					
19	May.02	49,303	10,718					
20	Jun.02	53,567	10,932					

Column B illustrates the entering of our HR measure, or nursing hours.

Column C illustrates the entering of our adjustment variable, or patient days for each month.

SECTION III: STEP-BY-STEP GUIDE TO MEETING THE STAFFING EFFECTIVENESS STANDARDS

Columns D and E

Once you've entered data for your HR measure (nursing hours for each month) in column B and the standardizing factor (patient days for each month) in column C, the ratio of your HR measure to the standardizing factor, or, in our case, nursing hours per patient days, is calculated in column D. If you are using our spreadsheet, column D already contains the formula for calculating nursing hours per patient day (the adjusted human resource measure) and should fill in automatically. This formula is simple: Nursing hours (column B) divided by patient days (column C) = nursing hours per patient day (column D). The next data item to enter is the clinical indicator, or, in our case, the patient satisfaction score from the nursing section of our hospital survey. These data are entered in column E of our spreadsheet. In the ten 20-bed patient care units of the hypothetical hospital, the patient satisfaction score for each month of the study period has been entered. See Screen Shot 9.

SCREEN SHOT 9

Column D calculates the ratio of our HR measure to the adjustment variable, or, in our case, nursing hours per patient days. This number is found by dividing the data in column B by column C.

Column E illustrates the entering of our clinical measure, or patient satisfaction.

	A	B	C	D	E	F	G	H
1	Unit of Analysis	Human Resource Variable	Adjustment Variable	Adjusted Human Resource Measure	Patient Outcome Variable	Rate of Patient Outcome to HR Measure		
2	Month	Nursing hours	Patient days	Nursing hours per patient day	Patient satisfaction	Ratio of patient satisfaction to nursing hours per patient day		
3	Jan.01	48,191	10,953	4.4	83%			
4	Feb.01	41,468	9,873	4.2	78%			
5	Mar.01	47,247	10.988	4.3	81%			
6	Apr.01	51,417	11,178	4.6	83%			
7	May.01	47,856	10,182	4.7	87%			
8	Jun.01	51,927	10,385	5.0	89%			
9	Jul.01	45,636	11,409	4.0	77%			
10	Aug.01	44,075	10,750	4.1	79%			
11	Sep.01	51,557	10,741	4.8	88%			
12	Oct.01	47,336	10,519	4.5	82%			
13	Nov.01	49,237	10,476	4.7	86%			
14	Dec.01	41,899	9,744	4.3	81%			
15	Jan.02	58,798	11,529	4.3	81%			
16	Feb.02	47,808	10,393	5.1	90%			
17	Mar.02	50,890	11,566	4,6	87%			
18	Apr.02	50,594	11,766	4.4	82%			
19	May.02	49,303	10,718	4.3	80%			
20	Jun.02	53,567	10,932	4.6	85%			

Section III: Step-By-Step Guide to Meeting the Staffing Effectiveness Standards

Column F

The final column in our spreadsheet—the ratio of patient satisfaction to nursing hours per patient day—should fill in automatically after you've entered data in columns B, C, and E. See Screen Shot 10. Column F shows patient satisfaction per 100 nursing hours per patient day. Remember, the calculation for this is to divide your clinical indicator (in our case, the patient satisfaction score in column E) by your HR indicator (in our case, nursing hours per patient day in column D) and multiply by a scaling factor of 100. (We are using 100 here to get a number higher than one, which is easier to work with.)

As noted earlier, our HR and clinical measures are probably correlated if the ratio does not change from month to month, meaning that the two indicators change together and are related. If the ratio is different from month to month, the HR and clinical indicators may not be correlated, meaning that when one changes, the other does not change proportionately.

SCREEN SHOT 10

Column F calculates the ratio of patient satisfaction to nursing hours per patient day.

	A	B	C	D	E	F	G	H
1	Unit of Analysis	Human Resource Variable	Adjustment Variable	Adjusted Human Resource Measure	Patient Outcome Variable	Rate of Patient Outcome to HR Measure		
2	Month	Nursing hours	Patient days	Nursing hours per patient day	Patient satisfaction	Ratio of patient satisfaction to nursing hours per patient day		
3	Jan.01	48,191	10,953	4.4	83%	18.86		
4	Feb.01	41,468	9,873	4.2	78%	18.57		
5	Mar.01	47,247	10.988	4.3	81%	18.84		
6	Apr.01	51,417	11,178	4.6	83%	18.04		
7	May.01	47,856	10,182	4.7	87%	18.51		
8	Jun.01	51,927	10,385	5.0	89%	17.80		
9	Jul.01	45,636	11,409	4.0	77%	19.25		
10	Aug.01	44,075	10,750	4.1	79%	19.27		
11	Sep.01	51,557	10,741	4.8	88%	18.33		
12	Oct.01	47,336	10,519	4.5	82%	18.22		
13	Nov.01	49,237	10,476	4.7	86%	18.30		
14	Dec.01	41,899	9,744	4.3	81%	18.84		
15	Jan.02	58,798	11,529	4.3	81%	18.84		
16	Feb.02	47,808	10,393	5.1	90%	17.65		
17	Mar.02	50,890	11,566	4.6	87%	18.91		
18	Apr.02	50,594	11,766	4.4	82%	18.64		
19	May.02	49,303	10,718	4.3	80%	18.60		
20	Jun.02	53,567	10,932	4.6	85%	18.48		

Section III: Step-by-Step Guide to Meeting the Staffing Effectiveness Standards

Analyzing your data

Selecting indicators, collecting data, and entering it into a spreadsheet are the foundations for gaining insight into the relationship between staffing and patient satisfaction (and, of course, meeting the JCAHO's standards)—regardless of the pair of HR and clinical indicators you have chosen. Data analysis is the next step in understanding staffing effectiveness. While sometimes perceived as daunting, data analysis is essential to design and implement effective change. And in fact, it is among the most creative aspects of performance improvement.

Data analysis is important both to overall patient satisfaction and to your efforts toward meeting the JCAHO's standards. As part of the staffing effectiveness standards, the JCAHO requires that collected data be analyzed and used to identify staffing effectiveness issues. JCAHO standard PI.4 takes that standard a step further by requiring you to use data to ensure that changes in process actually result in improvement.

Much as in for choosing your indicators and collecting data, JCAHO is nonprescriptive in its requirements for data analysis. You are required to examine possible relationships between staffing levels and patient satisfaction (or, more specifically, between an HR indicator and a clinical indicator), but you can choose to examine these relationships through a number of different methods. In our case, we're looking for a possible relationship between patient satisfaction and nursing hours per patient day.

Many data analysis concepts are common sense and executed easily. Other concepts will require using formulas and interpreting results from a statistical perspective. Wherever possible, we've simplified these concepts and provided the formulas for calculation within the companion spreadsheet. Before we take a more in-depth look at correlations, let's review statistical concepts and how they relate to our data.

Determining reasonability

Before you begin delving into your data, you'll want to conduct a reasonability scan—basically, checking to make sure all your data make sense. A reasonability scan involves reviewing volumes of activity or rates of occurrences. The data tabulated in the Excel spreadsheet should appear to have reasonable volumes and/or frequencies of events. Computing reasonability does not require a mathematical formula; is a common-sense assessment.

Unreasonable data does not automatically mean that your data are automatically incorrect. The unreasonableness could be attributed to several factors. These factors should be determined, and the variation should be explained.

Examples of the reasonability scan for the HR or clinical indicator data follow:

SECTION III: STEP-BY-STEP GUIDE TO MEETING THE STAFFING EFFECTIVENESS STANDARDS

- If you know that patient satisfaction is about 85% in a typical month, it is very unlikely that it would be 50% in a large unit with a good response rate. (Anything is possible, of course, if you receive only a few surveys back.)

- If you have a 450-bed hospital, you will not have more than 13,500 patient days in any month. There are about 30 days in a month, so your 450-bed hospital has a capacity of 450 x 30 = 13,500 patient days. If you are operating at 100% capacity, you might have 13,500 patient days. Many units, however, operate at 50–85% capacity, and this would translate into a volume of between 6,750–11,475 patient days—that is, less than 13,500, the quick calculation of 450 x 30.

Looking at our data in column C, you can see that our patient days are generally reasonable. Although patient days in the study period vary from one month to another, the patient days are within the 6,750–11,475 range that we mentioned above, except for three times in the first part of 2002 (January, March, and April). Patients stayed 11,766 days in April 2002, but only 9,744 days in December 2001. April 2002 with the most patient days in the study period has only about 20 percent more patient days than December 2001 with the fewest in the study period.

SCREEN SHOT 11

	A	B	C	D	E	F	G	H
1	Unit of Analysis	Human Resource Variable	Adjustment Variable	Adjusted Human Resource Measure	Patient Outcome Variable	Rate of Patient Outcome to HR Measure		
2	Month	Nursing hours	Patient days	Nursing hours per patient day	Patient satisfaction	Ratio of patient satisfaction to nursing hours per patient day		
3	Jan.01	48,191	10,953	4.4	83%	18.86		
4	Feb.01	41,468	9,873	4.2	78%	18.57		
5	Mar.01	47,247	10,988	4.3	81%	18.84		
6	Apr.01	51,417	11,178	4.6	83%	18.04		
7	May.01	47,856	10,182	4.7	87%	18.51		
8	Jun.01	51,927	10,385	5.0	89%	17.80		
9	Jul.01	45,636	11,409	4.0	77%	19.25		
10	Aug.01	44,075	10,750	4.1	79%	19.27		
11	Sep.01	51,557	10,741	4.8	88%	18.33		
12	Oct.01	47,336	10,519	4.5	82%	18.22		
13	Nov.01	49,237	10,476	4.7	86%	18.30		
14	Dec.01	41,899	9,744	4.3	81%	18.84		
15	Jan.02	58,798	11,529	4.3	81%	18.84		
16	Feb.02	47,808	10,393	5.1	90%	17.65		
17	Mar.02	50,890	11,566	4.6	87%	18.91		
18	Apr.02	50,594	11,766	4.4	82%	18.64		
19	May.02	49,303	10,718	4.3	80%	18.60		
20	Jun.02	53,567	10,932	4.6	85%	18.48		

- If your hospital has 10,000 patient days in a month, you are not likely to have more than 100,000 nursing hours in a month. The basis of this assumption is the number of nursing hours per patient day. On a med/surg care unit, you probably spend between four and six nursing hours per patient day. Multiplying this by 10,000 (patient days) yields 40,000 to 60,000 nursing hours.

If you are assessing ICUs, on the other hand, you may be applying significantly more nursing resources per patient, as many as 10 nursing hours per patient day. In this circumstance, you might expect to see 100,000 nursing hours associated with 10,000 patient days in a month.

The application of nursing resources to patient care will vary depending on the type of patient care unit. OB, rehabilitation, mental health, substance abuse, and geriatric acute care may have very different staffing strategies, particularly with respect to skill mix of patient care personnel. You will want to take this into account in your reasonability scan.

SECTION III: STEP-BY-STEP GUIDE TO MEETING THE STAFFING EFFECTIVENESS STANDARDS

Let's look back at our data. In column B, we've entered the total monthly nursing hours for each month. By reviewing the data entered in column B, you can see that the number of nursing hours accumulated during the study period varied between 41,468 in February 2001 and 58,798 in January 2002. The difference in nursing hours on these units may be a consequence of any number of factors (staff absence, different volumes of patients, etc.).

SCREEN SHOT 12

	A	B	C	D	E	F	G	H
1	Unit of Analysis	Human Resource Variable	Adjustment Variable	Adjusted Human Resource Measure	Patient Outcome Variable	Rate of Patient Outcome to HR Measure		
2	Month	Nursing hours	Patient days	Nursing hours per patient day	Patient satisfaction	Ratio of patient satisfaction to nursing hours per patient day		
3	Jan.01	48,191	10,953	4.4	83%	18.86		
4	Feb.01	41,468	9,873	4.2	78%	18.57		
5	Mar.01	47,247	10.988	4.3	81%	18.84		
6	Apr.01	51,417	11,178	4.6	83%	18.04		
7	May.01	47,856	10,182	4.7	87%	18.51		
8	Jun.01	51,927	10,385	5.0	89%	17.80		
9	Jul.01	45,636	11,409	4.0	77%	19.25		
10	Aug.01	44,075	10,750	4.1	79%	19.27		
11	Sep.01	51,557	10,741	4.8	88%	18.33		
12	Oct.01	47,336	10,519	4.5	82%	18.22		
13	Nov.01	49,237	10,476	4.7	86%	18.30		
14	Dec.01	41,899	9,744	4.3	81%	18.84		
15	Jan.02	58,798	11,529	4.3	81%	18.84		
16	Feb.02	47,808	10,393	5.1	90%	17.65		
17	Mar.02	50,890	11,566	4.6	87%	18.91		
18	Apr.02	50,594	11,766	4.4	82%	18.64		
19	May.02	49,303	10,718	4.3	80%	18.60		
20	Jun.02	53,567	10,932	4.6	85%	18.48		

Note: You will need to determine nursing hours per shift based on the specialty service of your unit, as well as the acuity index of your patients, so that nursing hours per shift can relate to actual staffing numbers.

Section III: Step-By-Step Guide to Meeting the Staffing Effectiveness Standards

- Nursing hours are not likely to vary by more than 20% from the lowest to the highest number of hours unless beds are closed for some study periods and not others. You may want to perform a preliminary calculation to determine this measure of reasonability. If, for example, on average, you have 330 of your 450 beds filled over a 30-day period (month) and your staffing ratio is four to five nurses per patient day, the range of nursing hours should be 39,600-49,500. Twenty percent below or above the average (48,823 nursing hours) would be about 39,000 nursing hours at the lower end and 58,600 nursing hours at the upper end.

  In the sample data in column B, you can see that this range was, in fact, exceeded. The highest number of nursing hours (58,798) is about 40% higher than the lowest number of nursing hours (41,468) across the 18 months. Exceeding the range could be attributed to several factors—staffing crisis, more intense patient demand for beds, etc. These special circumstances should be determined, and the variation should be explained. This is an example of seemingly unreasonable data that may be important analytically and operationally.

  The effect of the difference—that is, the effect of the difference of nursing hours on patient satisfaction—is, of course, what you hope to understand in studying the combination of your HR and clinical indicators.

Determining a reasonable range of values is important for analyzing your data. Some examples of reasonable ranges of values are as follows:

- Nursing hours per patient day are not likely to fall below two or three or to rise above six or seven on a med/surg unit. These ranges may vary, depending on the nursing demand in a specific unit. For example, in the ICU this range may be between eight and 12. Other ranges may be appropriate for patient care units providing other types of care (OB, nursery, pediatrics, rehabilitation, etc.).

  This range is on target for our data. In column D, nursing hours per patient day varied from 4.0 to 5.1 in the 18 months. You can see that higher patient days do not necessarily result in more nursing hours per patient day or vice versa. In fact, the lowest number of nursing hours per patient day (4.0) in July 2001 is not associated with the lowest number of nursing hours (41,468) or patient days (9,744). In fact, fewer patient days were recorded in December 2001, when the number of nursing hours was 41,899. Thus, the number of nursing hours per patient day was higher (4.3).

The month with the highest number of nursing hours per patient day is January 2002 at 5.1 nursing hours per patient day. There were more nursing hours in this month than any other month, but not more patient days.

Establishing control limits in patient satisfaction ratings

It is easiest to do a quick reasonability check by visualizing your data in a series of graphs. This also enables you to make a quick evaluation of the stability of the process through a technique called statistical process control. While a comprehensive review of statistical process control (SPC) and control limits is outside the scope of this book, we will include a few pointers that will help you ensure that your data are meaningful and appropriate for a staffing effectiveness analysis. (For more information about using SPC to analyze health care data, refer to the following reference: Raymond G. Carey and Robert C. Lloyd. *Measuring Quality Improvement in Healthcare: A Guide to Statistical Process Control Applications.* –(New York: Quality Resources, 1995)

For a rapid review of the data, you may want to use a line graph, also known as a run chart. When examining trends over time, a run chart is a useful tool, especially for ongoing monitoring and evaluation once you've implemented change, such as a new staffing plan intended to improve patient satisfaction. We will examine charts more closely in the presenting your data section, but we will look at them here for checking reasonability

Section III: Step-By-Step Guide to Meeting the Staffing Effectiveness Standards

You can generate a run chart that has months as its horizontal axis and patient satisfaction as its vertical axis. This is illustrated in Chart 1. Note that there is variation in the run chart. The lowest values occur in February 2001 (78%) and July 2001 (77%). There is a peak in January 2002 (90%).

Chart 1 illustrates the 18 months of patient satisfaction data displayed in a run chart or a control chart. The upper and lower control limits (95% and 72%, respectively) are three standard deviations (3 x 3.9%) away from the mean (83.6%) of the 18 data points. Control charts or run charts with control limits can be useful in determining whether an intervention was effective. (Mean and standard deviation are described in the next section of the workbook, which is about central tendencies and variability.)

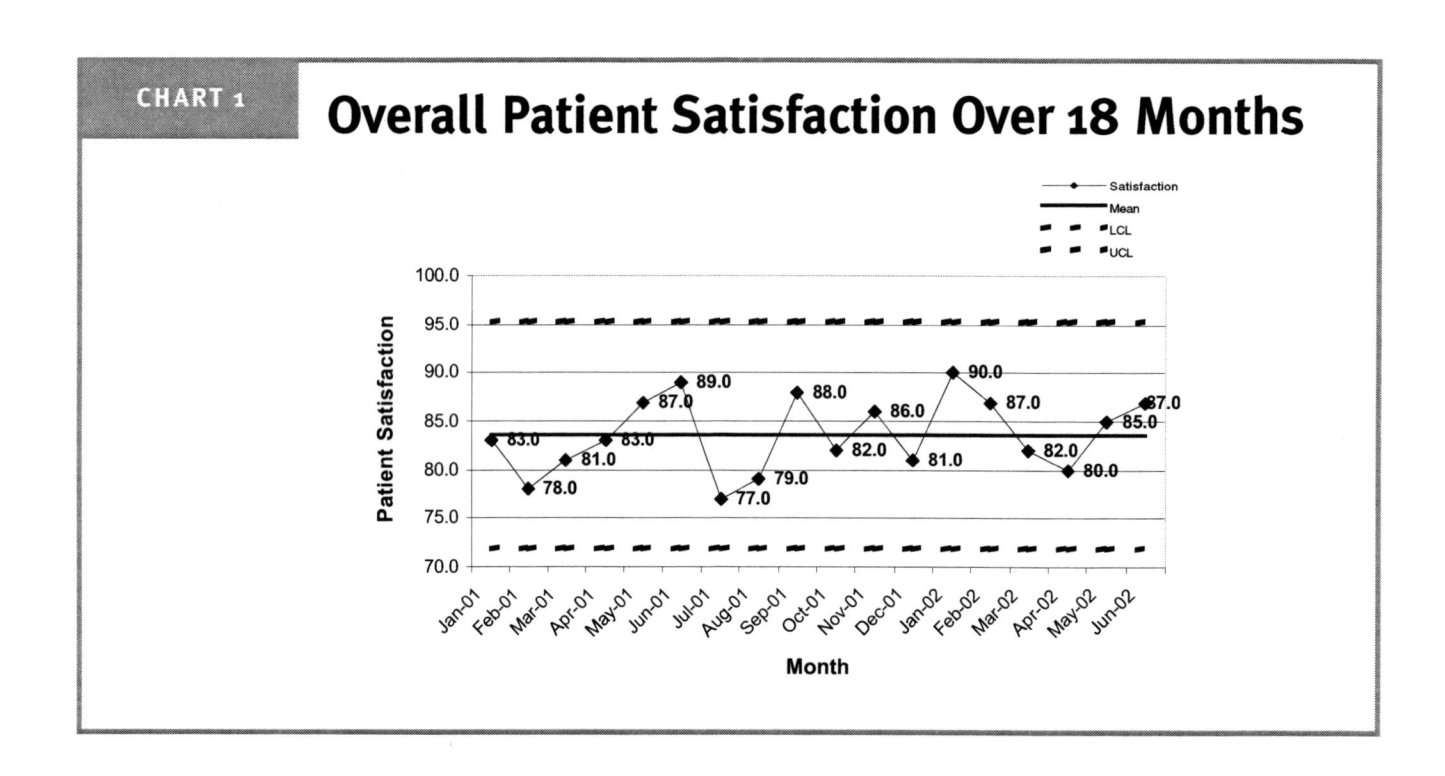

CHART 1

Overall Patient Satisfaction Over 18 Months

Section III: Step-By-Step Guide to Meeting the Staffing Effectiveness Standards

In reviewing historical performance, any data point that is more than three standard deviations above or below the mean represents an instance when the process may have been out of control. Once you have implemented an intervention or have changed processes in some way, you will look for changes in the control chart to confirm that you have achieved changes in outcome.

Any successive eight data points on the same side of the mean represent a significant change (a trend). So you'll be expecting a sustained improvement in patient satisfaction, following your patient satisfaction related intervention. If the change was implemented in July 2002, you will expect to observe patient satisfaction scores for eight successive months that are greater than 83.6%—the mean for the baseline period from January 2001 through June 2002.

How do you interpret the chart in Chart 1? While the data certainly fluctuate, they are moving within the upper and lower control limits, suggesting a stable process. Thus, you can feel comfortable that your process is stable, and you can move on to "drill down" factors that may influence the direction of change in the outcome (patient satisfaction).

Identifying "Data-Skewing" Outliers

In addition to reasonable ranges, you may also want to identify outliers whose inclusion in your data analysis significantly bias your results, to the extent that you cannot draw meaningful, action-oriented conclusions from the analysis. Once again, the JCAHO is non-prescriptive in its sampling requirements. You do not need to include all data (patients, units, etc.) to meet its requirements. From a statistics standpoint, what data you decide to include and exclude are critical to drawing reliable conclusions based on your data.

The following examples illustrate the importance of identifying outliers:

- One of your unit's beds was occupied by a patient who has not yet been discharged—that's 30 patient days (in a month) that must go into the denominator. When counting patient days, be sure to include patients who have not yet been discharged from the patient care unit. They have significant resource demand (nursing hours).

- One of the patients you discharged during the last month had stayed in the hospital for 227 days. If you are tracking one month of data, as we are, you should only count the days this month that the patient was on your unit.

  Note: If you are collecting data from your organization's finance systems, then you will not have to make these adjustments in patient days. The daily counting of the census will accommodate them.

- It is important to look at the number of survey responses before deciding whether to trim outliers from the data. If a unit received fewer than 30 surveys in a given period of time (e.g. a month), you will want to examine the data carefully. If it appears that the data follow fairly consistent and reasonable trends from prior and subsequent months, it is acceptable to retain the data for analysis. If there are fewer than 15 observations in one month or period, however, you will almost certainly exclude that unit's data from the monthly data set. Retain the data so that you can use it in a quarterly analysis, when you can accumulate more data.

Describing central tendencies and variability in a data set

Determining data and range reasonability, and identifying outliers, are part of the process of describing your study population. In order to analyze the data, however, you will also need to describe the study population with statistics that are calculated with mathematical formulas. Two common types of statistical description are measures of central tendency ("middleness") and measures of variability (variation in measurements from case to case).

Section III: Step-by-Step Guide to Meeting the Staffing Effectiveness Standards

So, why should you care about "middleness" and variation? You can use central tendency to evaluate staffing (HR) and outcome clinical indicator trends (over time), as well as to compare performance to external benchmarks. Is there a higher level of patient satisfaction when the hospital or unit is less busy? Has staffing practice changed, or is it different from external benchmarks?

A variation in measurements should be a marker for determining what really is a difference, as well as what may *appear* to be a change in performance but merely reflects normal fluctuations in the process. Clearly, you do not want to undertake significant efforts to correct a decline in performance unless you can demonstrate reliably that there was a decline. The most common problem in analyzing data is exactly this: paying too much attention to an ordinary "blip" in the data, thus wasting time and resources, or failing to recognize a meaningful trend in a timely fashion.

Variations in care are flags that a situation needs to be addressed or at least explained. While patient satisfaction levels across several units seem stable, is there a dramatic drop in one unit? If there are not enough observations to know whether patient satisfaction has fallen in that unit, you might conclude that the decline is just a chance occurrence. You will need to monitor satisfaction on this unit to determine whether there is a change in outcomes. (Beware of the famous "Hawthorn effect," in which the simple act of increasing your focus on that unit could result in changes in staffing patterns or staff behavior that could affect patient satisfaction results).

Before we delve into the statistical analysis, let's first cover the basics:

- **Variance:** Departure from the usual. Across 18 months, we observe that the patient satisfaction rating was 84% every month. Observation: There is no variability in the patient satisfaction rating over 18 months; hence, the statistical variance would be zero.

  Among the five med/surg units, on the other hand, patient satisfaction ratings for 18 months included three months at 81%, six months at 82%, five months at 83%, three months at 84%, and one month at 87%. Observation: There is variability—different patient satisfaction ratings were reported for the months in the study period.

  A statistical variance is derived from incorporating the ratings of care by patients into a formula. The result is an indication of the magnitude of the variance of patient satisfaction ratings over the 18 months.

- **Central tendency:** movement to the middle. In making numerous observations of a particular activity, the measurements will tend to cluster around one value: the middle. This is true of financial activity observations (like average costs or charges), nursing hours per month, and satisfaction levels on a patient care unit.

- **Mean:** the sum of values divided by the number of cases. For example, if your patient satisfaction ratings for five months are 79%, 82%, 80%, 85%, and 85%, you would find the mean (or the average) patient satisfaction rating by adding 0.79, 0.82, 0.80, 0.85, and 0.85, and dividing by 5.

$$\frac{.79+.82+.80+.85+.85}{5} = \frac{4.11}{5} = 0.82 \text{ or } 82\% = \text{mean}$$

- **Median:** the middle value, or central tendency, of all values being studied for a particular characteristic. For example, if you have five months of patient satisfaction ratings—79%, 82%, 80%, 85%, and 85%—the median would be 82% (the middle satisfaction rating in the set of satisfaction ratings that have been arranged in numerical order). In the case of the data in our spreadsheet, since there are 18 values for patient satisfaction and no one middle value, the median would actually be *half* of the sum of the 9th and 10th values, if the satisfaction ratings were ordered from least to greatest).

- **Mode:** the most frequently occurring value. For example, in a locked cabinet on the patient care unit, there are 15 aspirins, 13 ibuprofens, 10 Advil, and 11 Excedrin. Of the 49 tablets in the cabinet, there are more aspirin than any other category, so aspirin would be the mode of this distribution.

Using the above example of patient satisfaction ratings of 79%, 82%, 80%, 85%, and 85%, the mode would be 85%, because it appears the most frequently (i.e. two times vs. one time for the values 79%, 80%, and 82%).

- **Standard deviation:** the square root of the variance. Standard deviation is another measure of variability among data points. For example, if you have 18 months for which each month has an average of 5 nursing hours per day, there is no variation for nursing hours, and the standard deviation is zero.

But, if you have 18 months for which three months have an average of 4 nursing hours per patient day, six months have an average of 4.5 nursing hours per patient day, four months have an average of 5 nursing hours per patient day, two months have an average of 5.5 nursing hours per patient day, and three months have an average of 6 nursing hours per patient day, the standard deviation is 0.68 nursing hours per patient day. You won't have to calculate this yourself if you are using the companion spreadsheet. The formula for calculating standard deviation has already been entered.

What is a standard deviation of 0.68? What is 0.68's relevance? The mean of the number of nursing hours by month in the above example is 4.9 nursing hours per patient day. The standard deviation of 0.68 nursing hours per patient day is less than one-fifth of the mean (0.68 divided by 4.9 = 0.14), so this standard deviation is not very big. When the standard deviation approaches more than half of the mean (2.45 nursing hours per patient day in this example), there is a lot of variation among the values you are analyzing.

You will need to determine central tendency and variation (using the mean and median) before you can begin looking at the relationships between your staffing effectiveness indicators. Mean, median, and mode are used to begin examining relationships. The formulas for finding mean and median are quite simple to do yourself, but our spreadsheet will calculate them automatically once you've entered all the other data. Once you've calculated the mean and median, our spreadsheet will also calculate standard deviation. Rows 22–24 include the formulas for median, mean, and standard deviation.

Weighted Averages

You may have heard the term "weighted average." What is it, and when do we need to use it?

An average is simply computed by adding observations together and dividing by the number of observations, as we saw above. In our example, every patient's survey response is treated equally.

A weighted average is developed by treating each observation differently. Some are given more "weight" in the calculation than others. This is a useful technique when the "mix" of patients changes over time, and you want to make sure you are making comparisons consistently.

For example, let's suppose that you have patient satisfaction data for 12 months, but you have noticed two things: There are some differences in patient satisfaction among surgical, medical, and OB patients; and your mix of patients has changed so that OB is now a larger proportion of your patient population and surgical discharges are a smaller proportion. If you notice fluctuations in total average satisfaction, how do you make sure that you are studying patient satisfaction in a "fair" way, that you are not just seeing seasonal or population "mix" changes?

Here is an example of this problem, and how you might identify and resolve it:

1. Observe the hypothetical patient satisfaction data in Table 1. The "%" columns reflect the percentage of survey responses from each population. For example, in January, 35% of surveys came from medicine patients, 44% from surgical patients, and 21% from OB patients. The average score for each of the three groups is 83, 87, and 89, respectively.

SECTION III: STEP-BY-STEP GUIDE TO MEETING THE STAFFING EFFECTIVENESS STANDARDS

Weighted Averages (cont.)

TABLE 1

	Patient Satisfaction	Medical Patients		Surgical Patients		OB Patients	
	Overall Unweighted Average	% Survey Responses From Med. Patients	Average Satisfaction of Med. Patients	% Survey Responses From Surg. Patients	Average Satisfaction of Surg. Patients	% Survey Responses From OB Patients	Average Satisfaction of OB Patients
Jan.	86.0	35%	83	44%	87	21%	89
Feb.	86.6	35%	84	45%	87	20%	90
Mar	86.4	36%	85	45%	86	19%	90
Apr.	86.1	38%	83	46%	87	16%	91
May	86.5	37%	84	47%	88	16%	88
June	85.8	37%	85	44%	85	19%	89
July	86.4	36%	84	40%	87	24%	89
Aug.	86.5	33%	84	38%	86	29%	90
Sep.	87.4	32%	84	35%	87	33%	91
Oct.	87.0	33%	85	34%	86	33%	90
Nov.	87.2	33%	84	37%	87	30%	91
Dec.	86.7	32%	83	34%	86	34%	91
Total	86.5	35%	84.0	41%	86.6	25%	89.9

2. Graph the overall satisfaction average. From the trend, it appears that patient satisfaction is increasing.

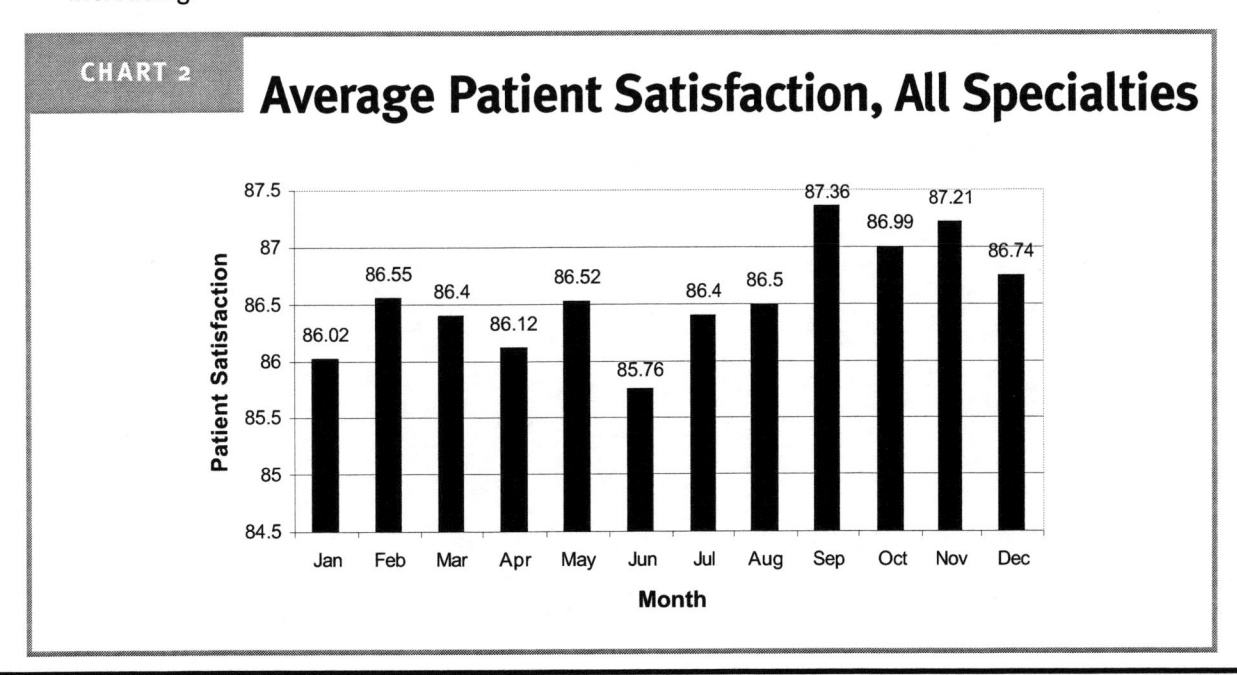

CHART 2

Average Patient Satisfaction, All Specialties

Month	Patient Satisfaction
Jan	86.02
Feb	86.55
Mar	86.4
Apr	86.12
May	86.52
Jun	85.76
Jul	86.4
Aug	86.5
Sep	87.36
Oct	86.99
Nov	87.21
Dec	86.74

INCREASING PATIENT SATISFACTION WITH STATISTICAL CORRELATION

SECTION III: STEP-BY-STEP GUIDE TO MEETING THE STAFFING EFFECTIVENESS STANDARDS

Weighted Averages (cont.)

3. Now you can check the "mix" of patients included in the data.

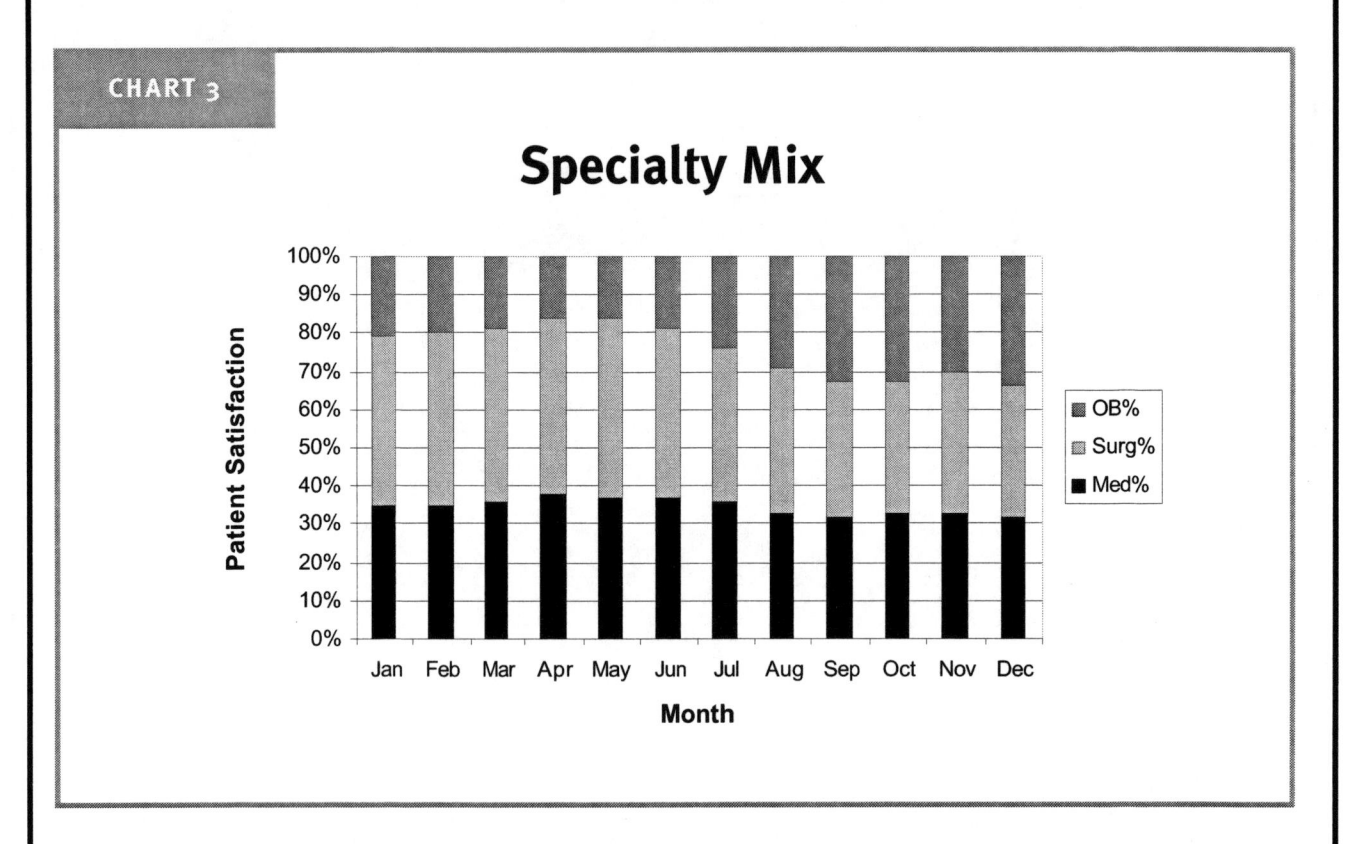

CHART 3

Specialty Mix

[Stacked bar chart showing monthly percentages from Jan to Dec, with Med%, Surg%, and OB% categories. Y-axis labeled "Patient Satisfaction" from 0% to 100%. X-axis labeled "Month".]

You notice immediately that OB is a larger proportion of the survey returns, surgery is smaller, and medicine is stable.

74   INCREASING PATIENT SATISFACTION WITH STATISTICAL CORRELATION

SECTION III: STEP-BY-STEP GUIDE TO MEETING THE STAFFING EFFECTIVENESS STANDARDS

Weighted Averages (cont.)

4. You want to check and see whether the three specialties tend to have different patient satisfaction patterns:

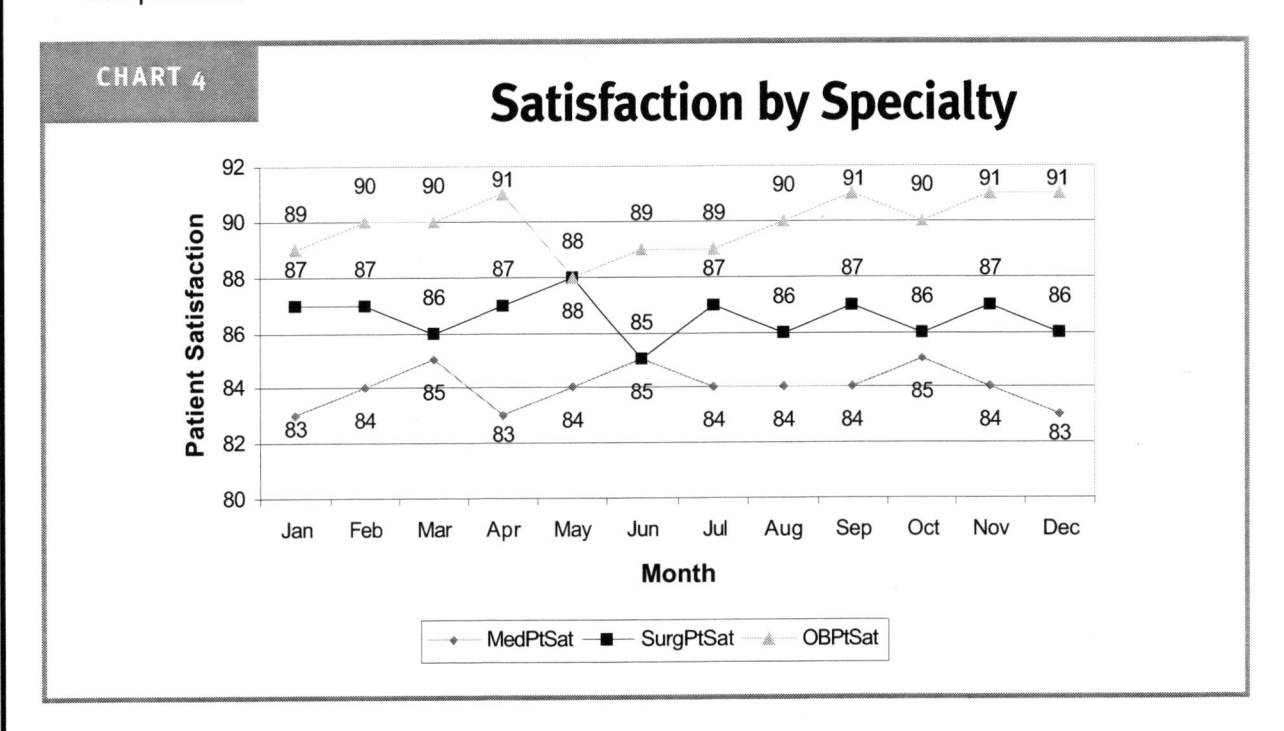

CHART 4

Satisfaction by Specialty

Month	MedPtSat	SurgPtSat	OBPtSat
Jan	83	87	89
Feb	84	87	90
Mar	85	86	90
Apr	83	87	91
May	84	88	88
Jun	85	85	89
Jul	84	87	89
Aug	84	86	90
Sep	84	87	91
Oct	85	86	90
Nov	84	87	91
Dec	83	86	91

You notice quickly that OB patients are the most satisfied, and this appears to be a consistent pattern. You also notice that OB and surgical patient satisfaction look pretty steady, and that medicine looks steady, although it declines in the last month or two.

You are concerned that the apparent improvement in satisfaction might be nothing more than the effect of more OB patients, so you decide that you need to recheck the analysis by removing the effects of the new "mix" change.

Weighted Averages (cont.)

5. You recompute the averages, but instead of using the actual percentage of patients each month, you "weight" each month's data by the *annual average percentage* "mix" of patients. For example, you weight medicine patient satisfaction at exactly 35% for every month, since this was its total percentage for the year. Surgery is weighted at 41% and OB at 25%.

TABLE 2

	Patient Satisfact.	Medical Patients		Surgical Patients		Obstetrics Patients		*Annual Average Mix*			Weighted Average
	Overall unweighted average	Med%	MedPt Sat	Surg%	SurgPt Sat	OB%	OBPt Sat	Med Mix	Surg Mix	OB Mix	
Jan.	86.0	35%	83	44%	87	21%	89	35%	41%	25%	86.1
Feb.	86.6	35%	84	45%	87	20%	90	35%	41%	25%	86.7
Mar.	86.4	36%	85	45%	86	19%	90	35%	41%	25%	86.6
Apr.	86.1	38%	83	46%	87	16%	91	35%	41%	25%	86.6
May	86.5	37%	84	47%	88	16%	88	35%	41%	25%	86.6
June	85.8	37%	85	44%	85	19%	89	35%	41%	25%	86.0
July	86.4	36%	84	40%	87	24%	89	35%	41%	25%	86.4
Aug	86.5	33%	84	38%	86	29%	90	35%	41%	25%	86.3
Sep.	87.4	32%	84	35%	87	33%	91	35%	41%	25%	86.9
Oct.	87.0	33%	85	34%	86	33%	90	35%	41%	25%	86.6
Nov.	87.2	33%	84	37%	87	30%	91	35%	41%	25%	86.9
Dec.	86.7	32%	83	34%	86	34%	91	35%	41%	25%	86.2
Total	86.5	35%	84.0	41%	86.6	25%	89.9				

SECTION III: STEP-BY-STEP GUIDE TO MEETING THE STAFFING EFFECTIVENESS STANDARDS

Weighted Averages (cont.)

6. On the basis of this "weighted" data set, you repeat the Average Patient Satisfaction, All Specialties graphic.

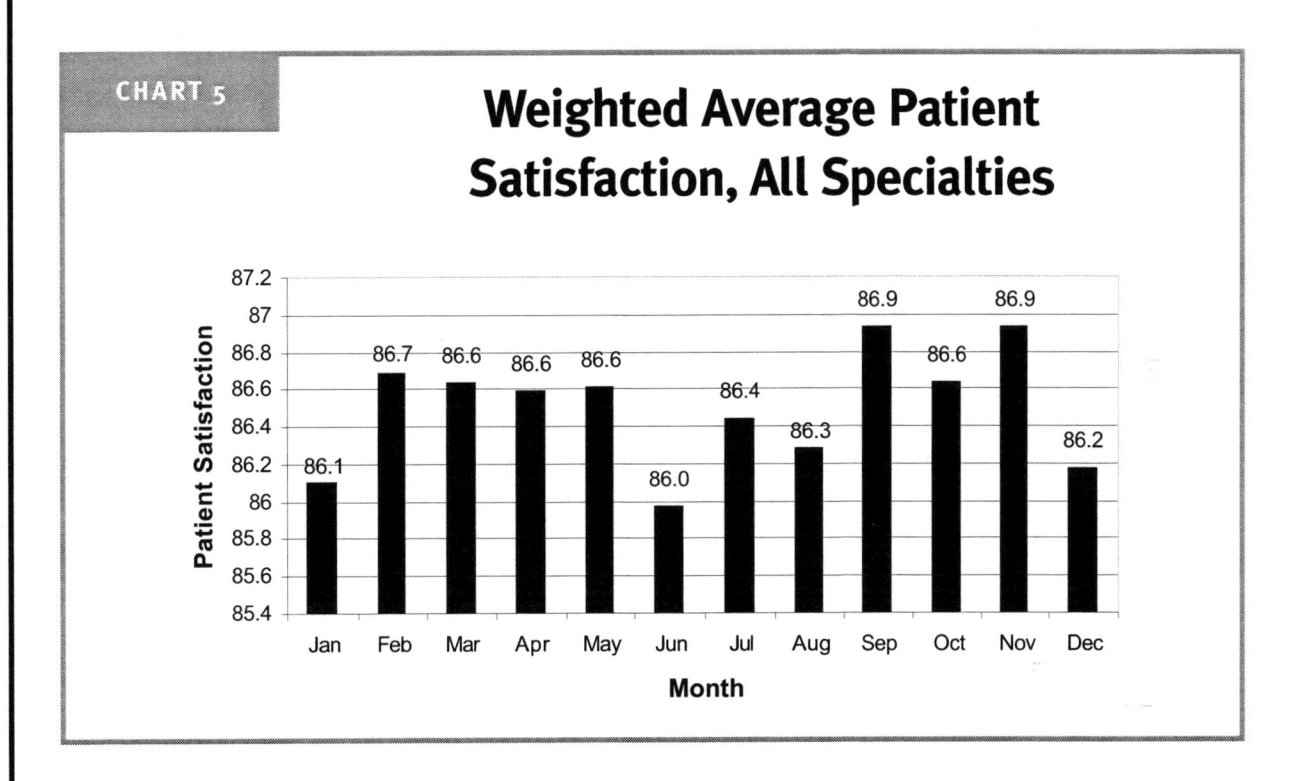

CHART 5

Weighted Average Patient Satisfaction, All Specialties

Month	Patient Satisfaction
Jan	86.1
Feb	86.7
Mar	86.6
Apr	86.6
May	86.6
Jun	86.0
Jul	86.4
Aug	86.3
Sep	86.9
Oct	86.6
Nov	86.9
Dec	86.2

And you observe that it does not appear that patient satisfaction has really increased, once you have removed the effect of the change in "mix" of patients.

You can compare the "raw" and "weighted" averages to see the effect of your "correction" to the data. You will notice that the two are different mainly in the last few months, when the mix of patients changed the most. There has been an improvement in patient satisfaction, but when the effect of the mix is removed, it appears that the improvement has been more modest than it first appeared.

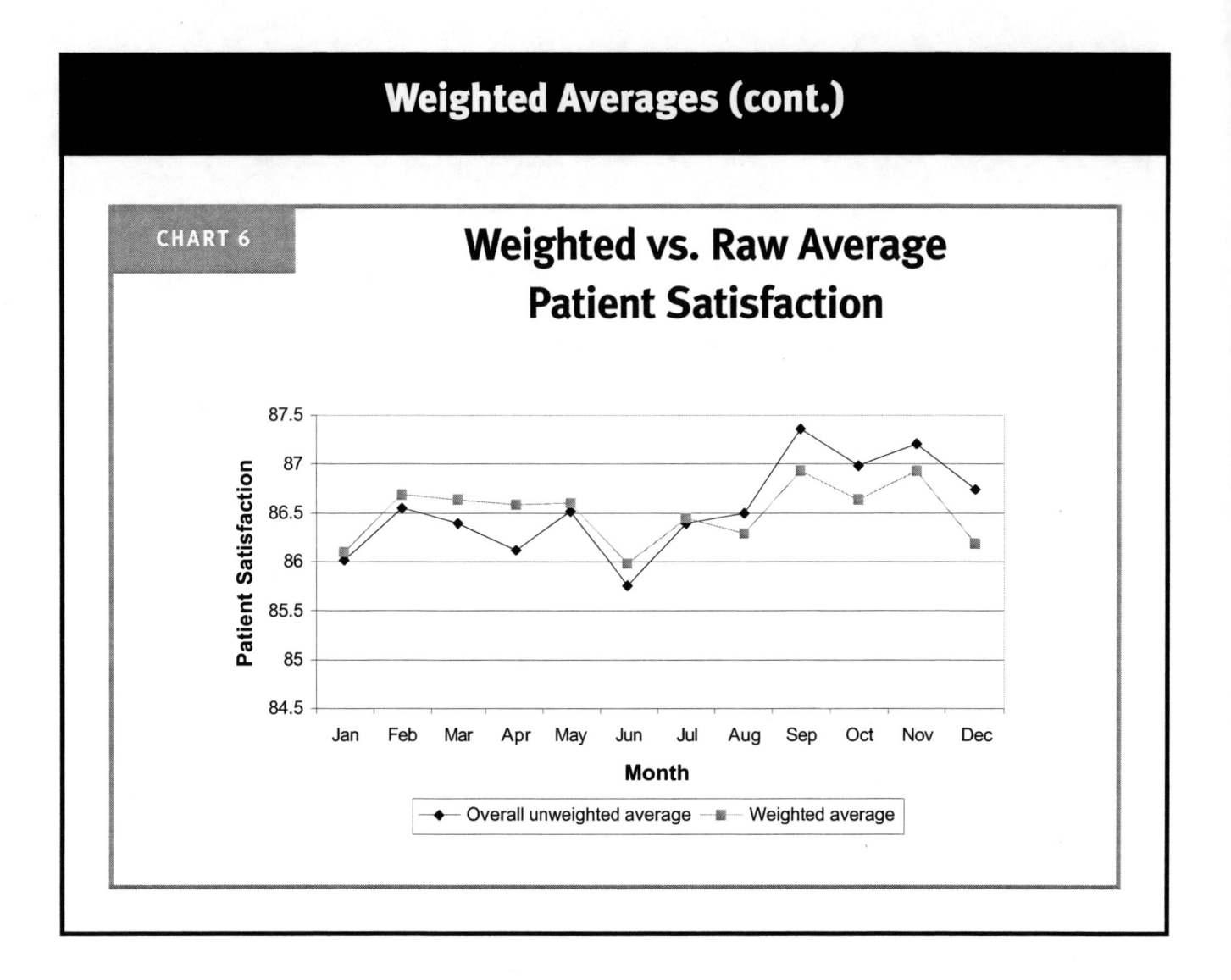

SECTION III: STEP-BY-STEP GUIDE TO MEETING THE STAFFING EFFECTIVENESS STANDARDS

Weighted Averages (cont.)

CHART 6

Weighted vs. Raw Average Patient Satisfaction

— Overall unweighted average — Weighted average

SECTION III: STEP-BY-STEP GUIDE TO MEETING THE STAFFING EFFECTIVENESS STANDARDS

Now let's return to the spreadsheet.

Row 22 in Screen Shot 12 contains an Excel formula that generates the mean value for a range of numbers in the spreadsheet. The data in columns B–F and rows 3-20 down, are added together and divided by 18 (the number of data points in each column).

SCREEN SHOT 12

	A	B	C	D	E	F	G	H
21								
22	Mean	48,823	10,783	4.53	83.6%	18.49		
23	Median	48,714	10,746	4.55	83.0	18.54		
24	Standard Deviation	4,169	570	0.31	3.9	0.476		
25	Correlation Coefficient Calculation	Nursing hours vs. overall satisfaction	Nursing hours vs. patient days	Overall satisfaction vs. patient days	nhppd vs. satisfaction			
26	Correlation Coefficient r	0.726	0.594	-0.070	0.96135			
27	r squared	0.527	0.353	0.005	0.924			

INCREASING PATIENT SATISFACTION WITH STATISTICAL CORRELATION

SECTION III: STEP-BY-STEP GUIDE TO MEETING THE STAFFING EFFECTIVENESS STANDARDS

The formula in row 23 calculates the median value for the range of numbers in each column of the spreadsheet. Based on the data entered in rows 3-20 of across B–F, the medians (or middle numbers) of those values appear in row 23, columns B through F, of the spreadsheet.

In our example, the means and medians are quite similar, suggesting that the values for the 18 patient satisfaction ratings are distributed normally. In our case, the mode is 87%, because it appears more than any other single value (three times). When no two values are the same, and you want to know what the mode is, you might group the data (as you would to generate a histogram) and identify a mode among the grouped data. For example, if we set up three ranges of nursing hours (40,000–47,999; 48,000–55,999; and 56,000–62,999), we see that there are more months where nurses worked 48,000–55,999 hours, specifically 9 of the 18 months. So, 48,000–55,999 nursing hours is the mode of the three categories.

SCREEN SHOT 13

	A	B	C	D	E	F	G	H
21								
22	Mean	48,823	10,783	4.53	83.6%	18.49		
23	Median	48,714	10,746	4.55	83.0	18.54		
24	Standard Deviation	4,169	570	0.31	3.9	0.476		
25	Correlation Coefficient Calculation	Nursing hours vs. overall satisfaction	Nursing hours vs. patient days	Overall satisfaction vs. patient days	nhppd vs. satisfaction			
26	Correlation Coefficient r	0.726	0.594	-0.070	0.96135			
27	r squared	0.527	0.353	0.005	0.924			

Section III: Step-by-Step Guide to Meeting the Staffing Effectiveness Standards

The formula in row 24 in our spreadsheet calculates the standard deviation of the data in columns B–F down rows 3-20. Remember that the standard deviation is the measure of variability of the 18 data items of each of the columns. Even if all columns have exactly the same standard deviation, however, the magnitude of the variability will not be the same necessarily. The magnitude of variability is actually found by looking at the ratio of the standard deviation—the value in row 24—to the mean—the value in row 22.

As you can see in our spreadsheet, less variability (i.e., smaller relative standard deviation) occurs in columns B–E, where the ratios of standard deviation to mean are 0.085, 0.053, 0.068, and 0.047, respectively. More variability (i.e., larger relative standard deviation) occurs where the ratios of standard deviation to mean are 0.50 or more. An outlier among the data points (for example, a month when the number of nursing hours was 90,000) is, in effect, an increase in variability and thus, an increase in standard deviation relative to the mean.

SCREEN SHOT 14

	A	B	C	D	E	F	G	H
21								
22	Mean	48,823	10,783	4.53	83.6%	18.49		
23	Median	48,714	10,746	4.55	83.0	18.54		
24	Standard Deviation	4,169	570	0.31	3.9	0.476		
25	Correlation Coefficient Calculation	Nursing hours vs. overall satisfaction	Nursing hours vs. patient days	Overall satisfaction vs. patient days	nhppd vs. satisfaction			
26	Correlation Coefficient r	0.726	0.594	-0.070	0.96135			
27	r squared	0.527	0.353	0.005	0.924			

Increasing Patient Satisfaction With Statistical Correlation

Section III: Step-by-Step Guide to Meeting the Staffing Effectiveness Standards

Making inferences about relationships

The JCAHO's staffing effectiveness standards require organizations like yours to undertake a process of using "inferential statistics"—a complicated-sounding term for a relatively simple concept. Using inferential statistics is basically the process of analyzing data to measure the strength and significance of the relationship among things that vary, or to predict outcomes based on experience or best judgment. For the staffing effectiveness standards, you are asked to examine possible relationships between staffing levels and patient outcomes (or, more specifically, between an HR indicator and a clinical indicator). In our case, we're looking for a possible relationship between patient satisfaction and nursing hours per patient day.

Several statistical methods address the significance of relationships, including the following:

- Simple examination of the ratio of the variables. In our spreadsheet, you will note that column F calculates a ratio of patient satisfaction to nursing hours per patient day. This is a simple and quick way to glance at the data to see if there are any apparent relationships. (The other methods described below will bring additional statistical rigor and tests of significance to any possible or apparent relationship.) Based on a quick scan of this column, there do not seem to be any obvious fluctuations in this ratio. Specifically, the smallest ratio, 17.65, occurs in February 2002, and it is not very different from the largest ratio, 19.27, which occurs in August 2001. The deviation from the ratio mean of 18.49 is less than 5% in either case, further evidence of a relatively constant ratio and thus a likely relationship between satisfaction ratings and nursing hours per patient day. Further analysis will be needed to see if there is a possible cause-and-effect relationship.

- Statistical correlation: uses the correlation coefficient r and determines if there is a correlation between two indicators. For example, you might use statistical correlation to determine if units with fewer nursing hours per patient day experience lower levels of satisfaction on average during the same period. **This is the statistical method we will be using**. *(Correlation is the appropriate statistical test to use when both of your indicator variables are continuous—that is, when they range from zero to 100 continuously, as in patient satisfaction.)*

- Chi square: determines whether the distribution of one value is contingent upon another value. For example, you might use chi square to determine if units whose nursing hours per patient day are greater than the median number of nursing hours per patient day receive more "top box" (highest possible score) ratings of patient satisfaction than units whose nursing hours per

Section III: Step-by-Step Guide to Meeting the Staffing Effectiveness Standards

patient day are lower than the median. *(Chi square is the appropriate statistical test to use when your indicator variables are "interval" data—that is, when they represent discrete scores, such as number of patients awarding the "best" score on the survey.)*

- T-test: determines whether two group measures are different. For example, you might use a t-test to compare the monthly patient satisfaction scores on Unit 1 in the 12 months before and after revising your staffing plan.

- Regression equation: predicts the value of a measure from the value of another measure (or several measures). The regression equation is developed using historical data. The measures used in the development are selected on the basis of the likelihood of a clinical and/or operational relationship among measures. The result is an equation that can be used to calculate the expected value of an outcome measure, knowing the value of the related measure. For example, you might use a regression equation to predict that as nursing hours *per patient day* increase, patient satisfaction will also increase.

Because the JCAHO's standards require only that you to look for a relationship, you could use any of the above tests to determine the significance of your indicators' relationship. For our purposes, we are looking to see if there is a correlation between patient satisfaction and nursing hours per day that reflects our hypothetical hospital's staffing effectiveness; therefore, we'll be evaluating the strength of our relationship by calculating the correlation coefficient *r*.

When There Is No Correlation/Statistical Relationship

If there is no relationship, does this mean that you are out of compliance with the JCAHO's requirements?

If you perform the analyses described here, you may discover that, in fact, the measures you have chosen do not appear to have a statistical relationship, suggesting that staffing is not a factor in influencing your clinical outcome (e.g., patient satisfaction). You will need to take the following steps:

1. From a compliance perspective, even if you do not find a correlation between your indicators, you have met the JCAHO's intent by undertaking the process of looking at the relationship.

2. Perform technical quality control. Ensure that you have, in fact, collected and used the proper measures, have correlated them correctly, etc.

3. Use your QI committee or appropriate oversight group to review and reflect on the data. Engage the group in discussion of the original hypothesis, and what the lack of correlation means. What are other possible staffing factors that may affect patient satisfaction? What are some possible data problems to address—for example, is there a lower response rate in a particular area?

4. Consider with your QI committee whether you should "drill down" to another level. Should you repeat the analysis for major specialties individually, rather than just performing it hospital-wide (e.g., medical units, surgical units, OB, pediatrics, etc.)? Now that you have the methodology clarified, this will be considerably easier the second time.

5. You may want to challenge the group to consider a different measure that you believe may influence patient satisfaction. Instead of *nursing hours per patient day*, it may be desirable to look at *agency hours as a percentage of nursing hours per day* or some other, more sophisticated measure.

6. It is essential that you continue to examine staffing and clinical measures, both for your own QI program and for JCAHO compliance. Thus, even in the absence of a correlation for one set of data, your work is not complete; you need to move ahead by refining your measures, or perhaps creating a new set of measures.

SECTION III: STEP-BY-STEP GUIDE TO MEETING THE STAFFING EFFECTIVENESS STANDARDS

So, how will you know if a correlation exists between your indicators?

The result of a statistical correlation is a number known as the correlation coefficient, which is often represented as *r*. The formula for finding *r* is complex, but your Excel spreadsheet should automatically calculate it for you. The range of *r* is between –1.0 and +1.0. The closer *r* is to –1.0 or +1.0, the greater the strength of the relationship. The closer *r* is to zero, the weaker the strength of the relationship. If *r* is exactly +1.0 or –1.0, it's a perfect correlation. If *r* is zero, on the other hand, there's no correlation at all.

Negative values of *r* mean that the indicators are related reciprocally—that is, as one indicator takes on larger values, the other takes on smaller values, and vice versa. An example of a reciprocal relationship might be that as the number of nursing hours decreases, the number of patient complaints (or satisfaction ratings in the "very poor" range) increases.

Positive correlations, on the other hand, imply a direct relationship—that is, as the value of one indicator increases, the value of the second one increases as well. For example, as the number of nursing hours increases, average patient satisfaction increases.

Correlation Coefficient *r*

If *r* is...	Then the relationship of the indicators or variables is...
1.0	Perfect positive relationship: as one goes up, the other goes up
Between 1.0 and 0.5	Strong positive relationship: as one goes up, the other usually goes up
Between 0.5 and 0	Weak positive relationship: as one goes up, the other tends to go up, but it is not consistent or reliable
Between 0 and -0.5	Weak negative or inverse relationship: as one goes up, the other tends to go down
Between -0.5 and -1.0	Strong negative or inverse relationship: as one goes up, the other usually goes down
-1.0	Perfect negative or inverse relationship: as one goes up, the other goes down

INCREASING PATIENT SATISFACTION WITH STATISTICAL CORRELATION

A related calculation is r^2, or the correlation coefficient times itself. This number is useful for several reasons: First, it is easy to work with because it has a narrower range, zero to +1.0; second, it is never negative.

r^2 Coefficients

If r^2 is...	The relationship of the indicator variables is...
Close to 1.0	a near perfect relationship: as one moves, the other moves quite consistently (may be positive or negative)
Between 0.5 and 1.0	a strong relationship: as one moves, the other tends to move reliably (may be positive or negative)
Between 0.25 and 0.5	probably a reliable relationship (the underlying correlation or r is at least 0.5): as one moves, the other tends to move (may be positive or negative)
Below 0.25	probably not a reliable relationship

The r^2 will not tell you, however, if that relationship is reciprocal (negative or inverse) or direct (positive). Often in data analysis, it is most important, initially, to know whether or not a relationship exists. A simple graph will confirm the direction of the relationship.

Section III: Step-by-Step Guide to Meeting the Staffing Effectiveness Standards

The r^2 can be computed automatically and displayed in x-y charts in Excel. As you'll see in the presentation section, x-y charts allow you to plot two measures on the same chart, giving you insight into the relationship between measures, rather than just providing information about separate indicators, as bar charts and histograms do.

Example: The Importance of Standardizing Data

This example further emphasizes the relevance and importance of standardizing data. Consider this scenario, which uses a different set of data points from those in the hypothetical hospital described above and from those in the spreadsheet accompanying this book:

You compare total paid nursing hours to average patient satisfaction. Your hypothesis is that more nursing hours should be related to higher patient satisfaction.

To your amazement, you notice that it seems that they are *inversely* related. As nursing hours increase, patient satisfaction *decreases*.

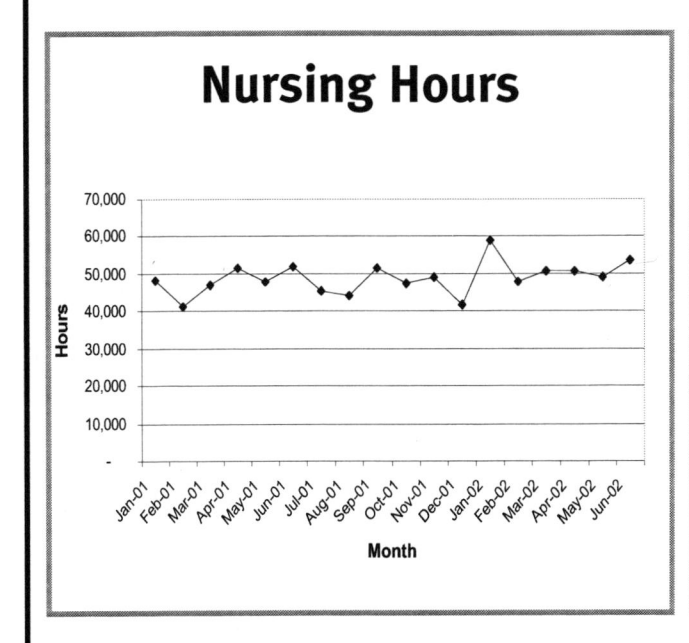

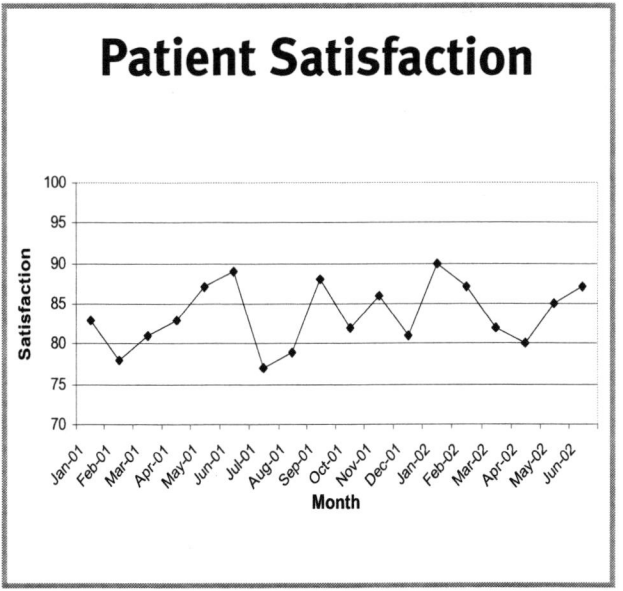

Example: The Importance of Standardizing Data (cont.)

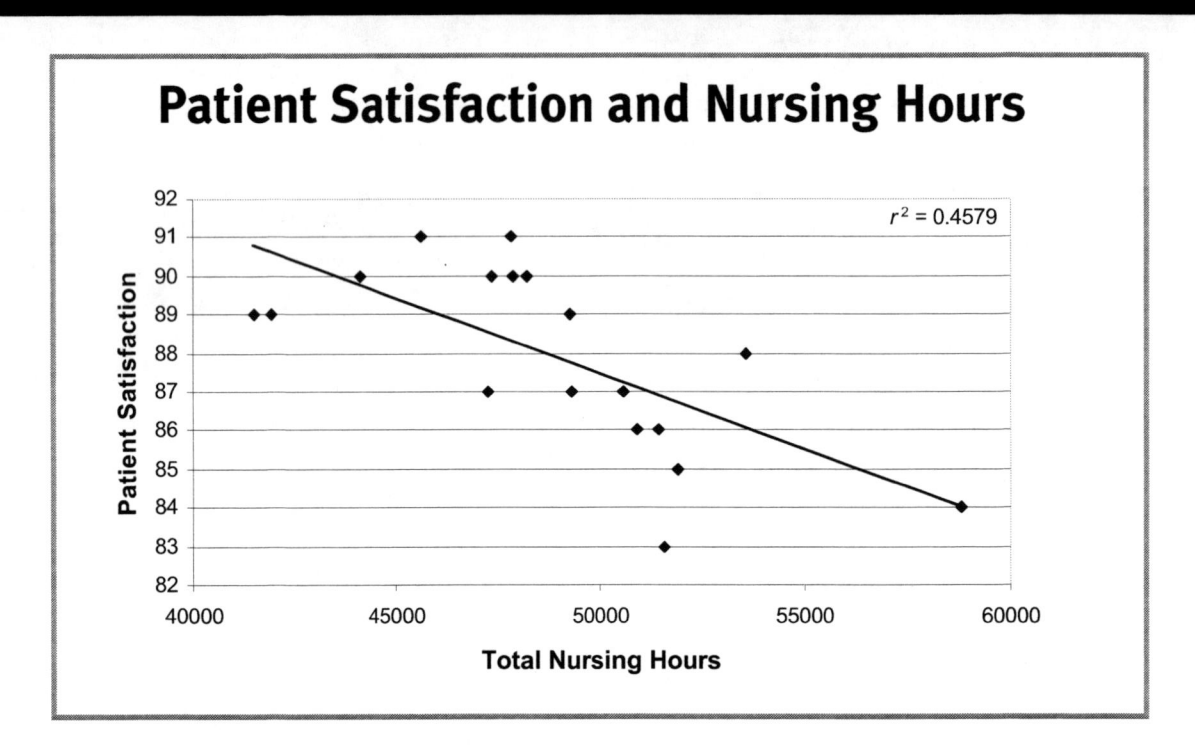

Patient Satisfaction and Nursing Hours

$r^2 = 0.4579$

With an r^2 of 0.46, you are convinced that there is a meaningful *negative* relationship between the two indicators, nursing hours and patient satisfaction. (Recall that an r^2 of 0.46 means that the two variables are correlated at about 0.68, a strong relationship.)

As you review the data with your committee, someone comments that the census was very high for several months. The unit nurse manager (who may be feeling a bit defensive) reminds the committee that she has budget flexibility to add staff if the census is high. She says, however, that she can't understand how satisfaction could *decline* with *more* nursing staff.

You go back to the data and realize that you have not adjusted nursing hours for the number of patient days—i.e., the high or low census. In other words, this graph shows you simply that satisfaction was lower when total nursing hours in the hospital were lower. This could mean that satisfaction was lower on low-census days. Or it could mean that satisfaction was lower when there were not enough nursing hours for the census. You do not have enough information at this point to determine which of these is correct, or whether there are still other hypotheses or factors to consider.

Section III: Step-by-Step Guide to Meeting the Staffing Effectiveness Standards

Example: The Importance of Standardizing Data (cont.)

You form a new hypothesis: When more nursing hours are available *for each patient* present on the unit *(i.e., nursing hours per patient day)*, patient satisfaction with nursing care should be higher.

You recalculate, and instead of comparing patient satisfaction to nursing hours, you compare it to *nursing hours per patient day*.

Month	Nursing hours	Patient days	Nursing hours per patient day	Patient Satisfaction
Jan 01	48,191	10,000	4.8	0.9
Feb 01	41,468	9,873.35	4.2	0.89
Mar 01	50,890	11,566	4.4	0.86
Apr 01	50,594	11,766	4.3	0.87
May 01	49,303	11,100	4.4	0.87
Jun 01	51,927	12,300	4.2	0.85
Jul 01	45,636	10,000	4.6	0.91
Aug 01	44,075	9,900	4.5	0.9
Sep 01	51,557	12,700	4.1	0.83
Oct 01	47,336	10,519	4.5	0.9
Nov 01	49,237	10,476	4.7	0.89
Dec 01	41,899	9,744	4.3	0.89
Jan 02	58,798	13,400	4.4	0.84
Feb 02	47,808	10,393	4.6	0.91
Mar 02	47,247	10,987.7	4.3	0.87
Apr 02	51,417	12,000	4.3	0.86
May 02	47,856	10,182.1	4.7	0.9
Jun 02	53,567	12,500	4.3	0.88

Increasing Patient Satisfaction With Statistical Correlation

Example: The Importance of Standardizing Data (cont.)

The resulting data confirm that satisfaction is actually correlated directly with nursing hours, *when adjusted for patient volume (e.g., per patient day)*. That is, when nursing hours per patient day increase, patient satisfaction increases. The r^2 value of 0.465 indicates a reasonably consistent relationship, with r being the square root of r^2, or 0.68.

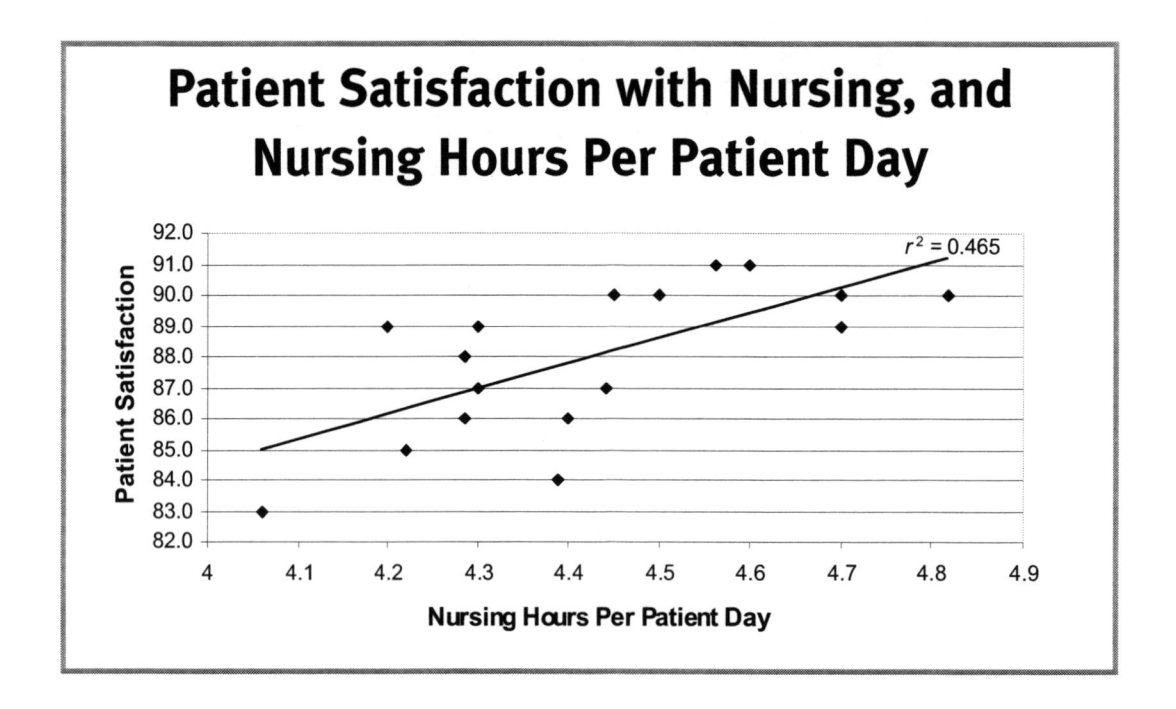

Patient Satisfaction with Nursing, and Nursing Hours Per Patient Day

$r^2 = 0.465$

SECTION III: STEP-BY-STEP GUIDE TO MEETING THE STAFFING EFFECTIVENESS STANDARDS

In Screen Shot 15 below (which includes the calculations for mean, median, and standard deviation), there are calculations for measuring the relationship between the HR indicator and the clinical indicator. The section appears in rows 25–27 across columns A–E. Column A contains a brief description of the information that appears in columns B–E. Row 25 contains the description of the relationship being tested. The formula in row 26 calculates the r. The formula in row 27 calculates r^2.

SCREEN SHOT 15

	A	B	C	D	E	F	G	H
21								
22	Mean	48,823	10,783	4.53	83.6%	18.49		
23	Median	48,714	10,746	4.55	83.0	18.54		
24	Standard Deviation	4,169	570	0.31	3.9	0.476		
25	Correlation Coefficient Calculation	Nursing hours vs. overall satisfaction	Nursing hours vs. patient days	Overall satisfaction vs. patient days	nhppd vs. satisfaction			
26	Correlation Coefficient r	0.726	0.594	-0.070	0.96135			
27	r squared	0.527	0.353	0.005	0.924			

INCREASING PATIENT SATISFACTION WITH STATISTICAL CORRELATION

SECTION III: STEP-BY-STEP GUIDE TO MEETING THE STAFFING EFFECTIVENESS STANDARDS

Chart 7 illustrates the relationship between nursing hours and patient satisfaction (column B) in our hypothetical hospital data set.

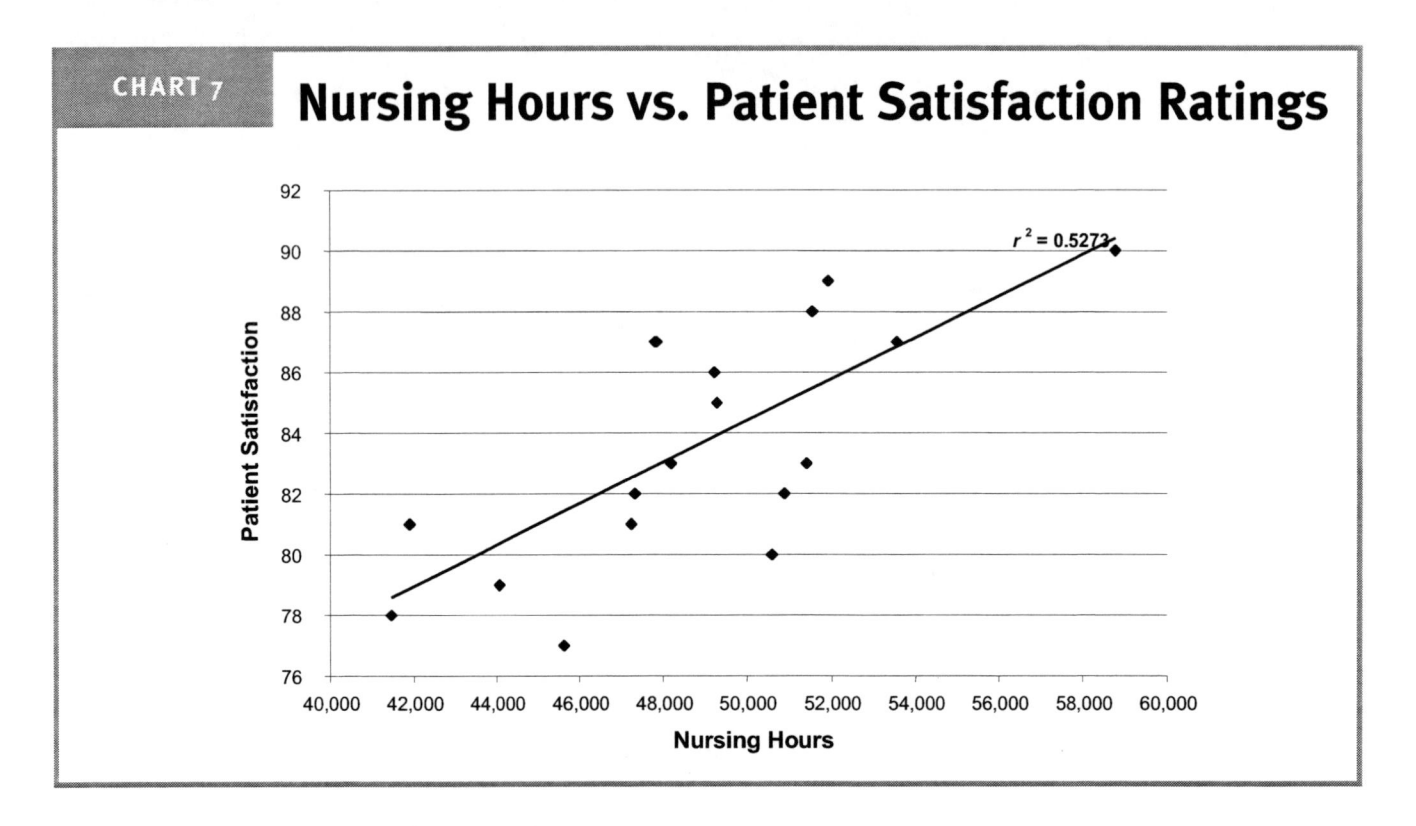

CHART 7: Nursing Hours vs. Patient Satisfaction Ratings

$r^2 = 0.5273$

The relationship between nursing hours and patient satisfaction appears to be mildly related in these data. The r^2 of 0.5273 confirms that there is a strong association between these data. The related correlation coefficient r for an r^2 of 0.5273 is 0.7262.

If you examine the chart, you will notice that the observations (data points) do not all fall exactly on the r^2 line. If they did, we would have a perfect relationship (1.0). What you can see is that they move in a similar direction. It certainly appears, glancing casually, that an increase in one variable is associated with an increase in the other.

It is not until we compute the r or r^2 statistics, however, that we can confirm our intuitive sense that there is a relationship and quantify the reliability of that relationship.

In this case, if we know how many nursing hours were worked in a given unit in a given month, we can still predict to a limited degree the level of patient satisfaction in that unit. We have not adjusted, however, for patient *volume* in the data yet.

SECTION III: STEP-BY-STEP GUIDE TO MEETING THE STAFFING EFFECTIVENESS STANDARDS

Why do we need to adjust for volume? Consider your conclusion thus far: **Patient satisfaction increases when nursing hours increase.**

This conclusion does not meet a "reasonability" test. Any experienced manager will challenge such a conclusion immediately, pointing out that you can't just examine hours unless you know how many patients were receiving care at a given time. And leaders are sure to note that it is not possible, reasonable, or responsible to simply increase nursing hours without limit; you need to know what activities you are staffing.

So the question is: *What is the right staffing level, given patient volumes, to optimize patient satisfaction?*

First, let's see how you are doing at staffing to volume. Do you have a consistent pattern of adjusting your staffing to patient days?

Chart 8 illustrates the relationship between nursing hours and patient days (column C). Here, we see strong positive correlation (r and r^2 nearer to 1.0 than zero) between nursing hours and patient days.

CHART 8

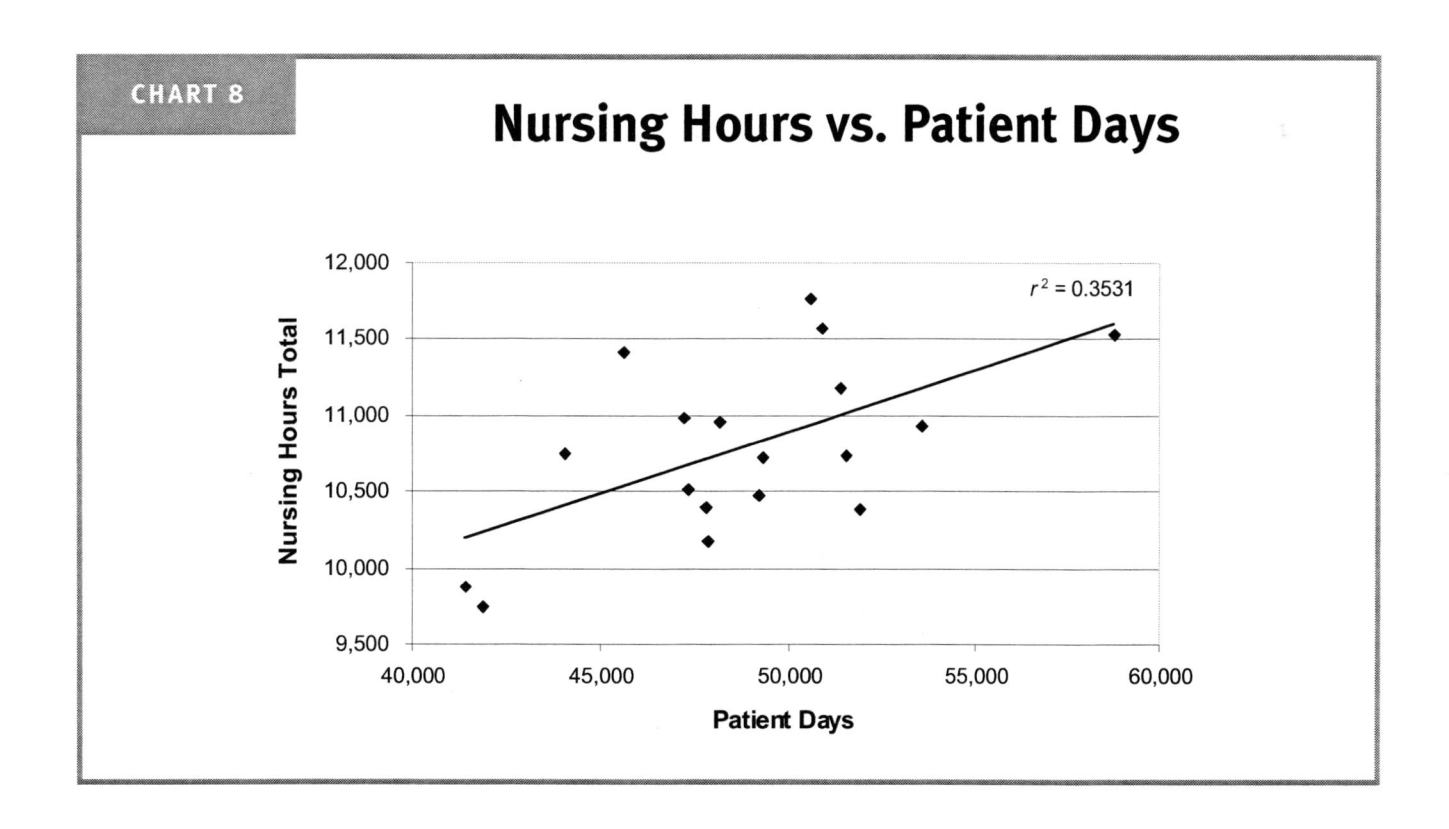

Nursing Hours vs. Patient Days

$r^2 = 0.3531$

The discussion of the relationship between nursing hours and patient satisfaction applies to the relationship between nursing hours and patient days. Among homogeneous types of patient care units (whether med/surg, ICUs, or geriatric care units), the correlation between nursing hours and patient days is expected to be high.

All this means is that your management team is doing a good job of staffing according to volume. Your budget and financial management processes will provide the discipline to make sure that staffing ratios are kept within target ranges. If they vary from the plan, your staffing effectiveness analysis will help you to determine whether those variances were helpful in delivering desirable clinical outcomes. For instance, if a unit overstaffs consistently (according to budget) but can show significantly higher patient satisfaction statistically, you will have a data set to assist in the decision of what the *right* budget numbers should be.

The JCAHO's staffing effectiveness standards anticipate specifically that the results of your analysis *will* be used to inform and enrich staffing decisions.

If you do not find a strong correlation (r closer to zero than 1.0) among homogeneous patient care units, you may want to investigate the source of the dissimilarity. Inaccurate data is a potential source, whether reported inconsistently or entered into the spreadsheet incorrectly. Or different interpretations of patient management policies among nursing managers have resulted in different staffing patterns. While this is not, in itself, a focus of the staffing effectiveness analysis, it is important to understand your staffing patterns to make sense of the outcomes that you are analyzing (in our case, patient satisfaction).

SECTION III: STEP-BY-STEP GUIDE TO MEETING THE STAFFING EFFECTIVENESS STANDARDS

Chart 9 illustrates the relationship between patient satisfaction and patient days (column D). The scatterplot of these two variables appears to be quite random, and the r^2 confirms that there is no statistical relationship ($r^2 < .005$).

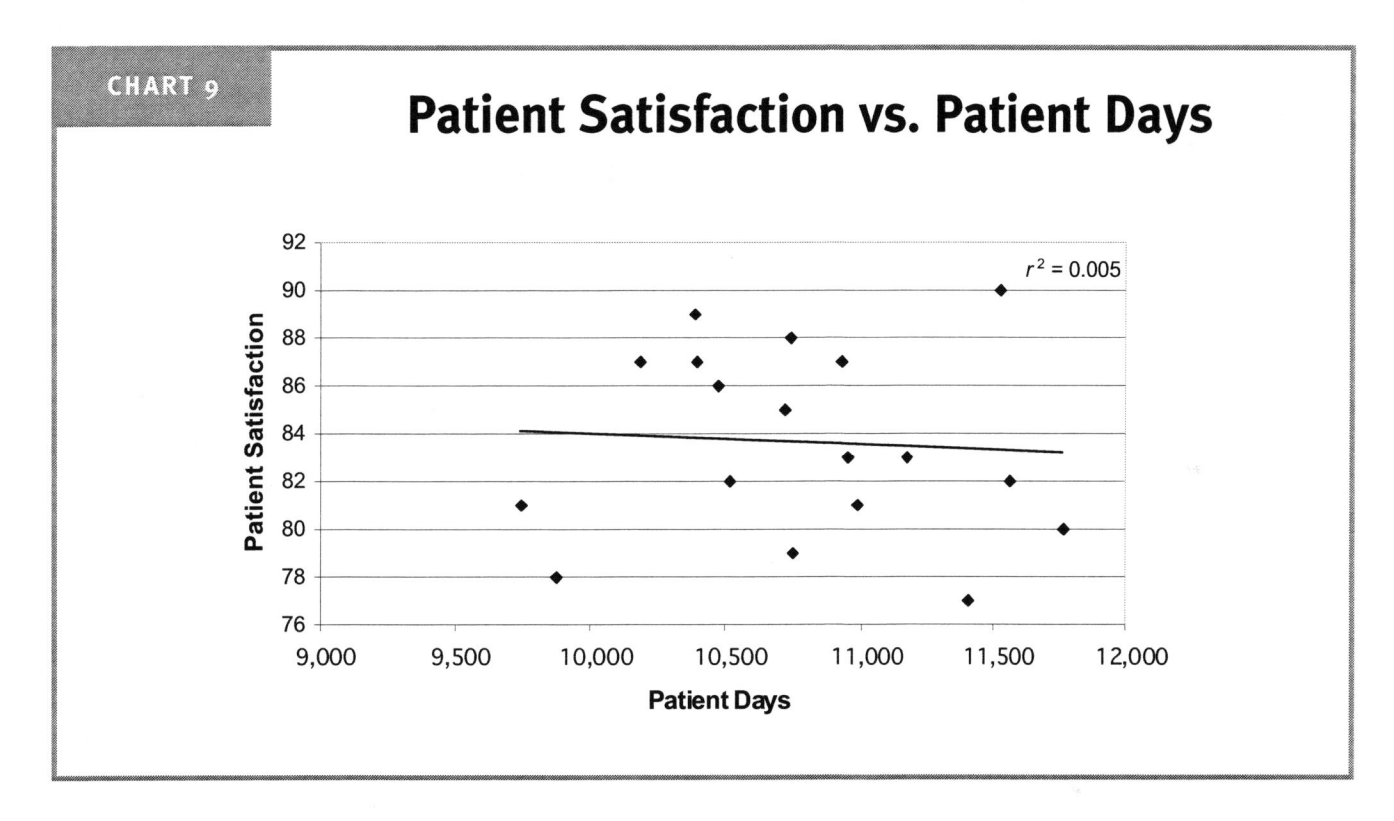

CHART 9

Patient Satisfaction vs. Patient Days

$r^2 = 0.005$

In operational terms, this is important. To management, it means that we cannot conclude simply that being busy is related directly to patient satisfaction results. Clearly, there is another intervening variable (and our hypothesis is that nurse staffing is that variable).

Section III: Step-by-Step Guide to Meeting the Staffing Effectiveness Standards

The last column in the section of the spreadsheet—column E—tests the relationship between nursing hours *per patient day* and satisfaction with nursing care. This relationship is the essence of determining staffing effectiveness in our hypothetical hospital with the pair of measures we have selected.

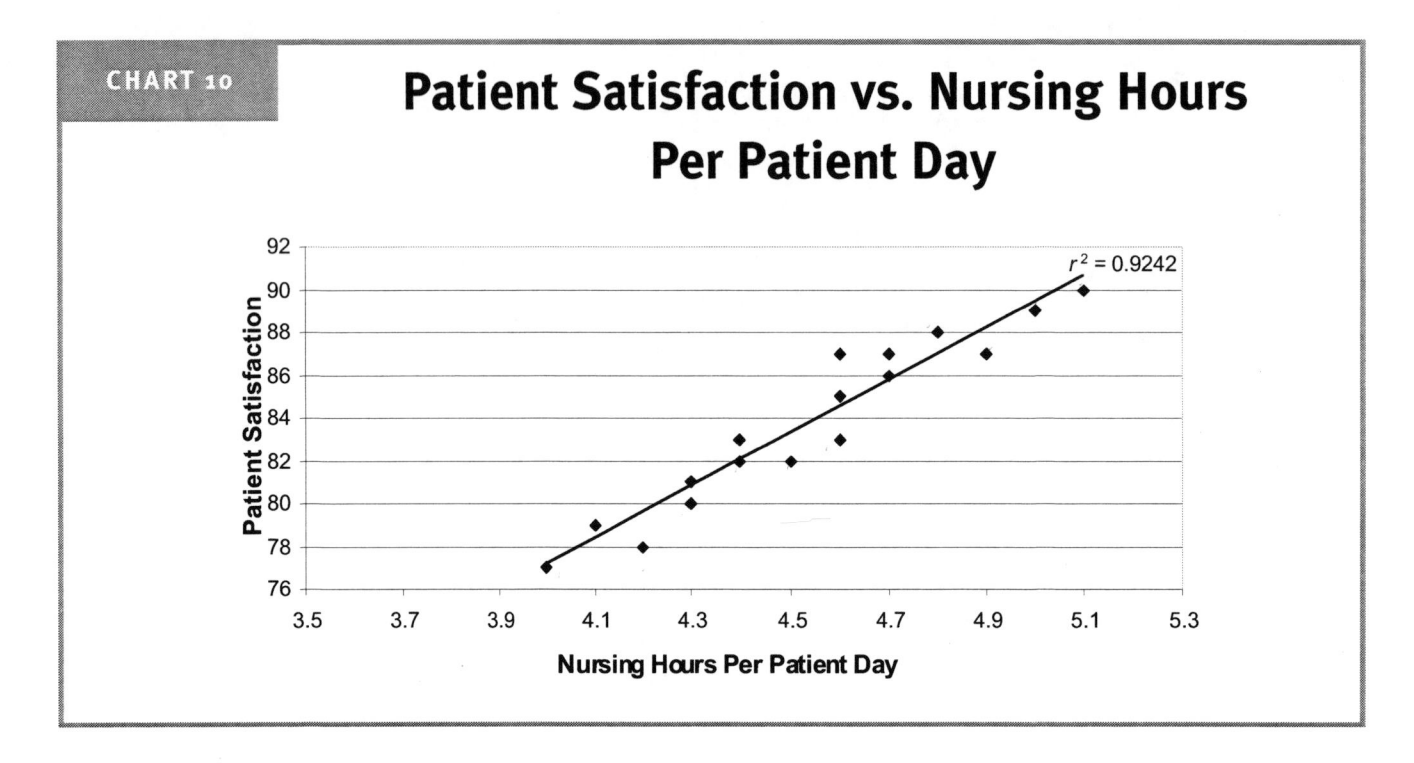

CHART 10

Patient Satisfaction vs. Nursing Hours Per Patient Day

$r^2 = 0.9242$

(Scatter plot with Patient Satisfaction on y-axis ranging from 76 to 92, and Nursing Hours Per Patient Day on x-axis ranging from 3.5 to 5.3)

As you can see, the relationship between nursing hours per patient day and satisfaction is an extremely powerful one. The r^2 is 0.9242, an almost perfect relationship. The conclusion for management is that **as standardized nursing hours per patient day increase, patient satisfaction can be expected to increase reliably.**

Many staffing effectiveness analyses will produce meaningful correlations but not reach this very strong level. This is to be expected, since many factors are involved in meeting patients' needs for an acceptable and satisfactory experience in the hospital.

How can you make sense of *your* correlation data?

Absence of a strong relationship (*r* value near zero) would suggest that factors other than staffing might be driving patient satisfaction. This could be the result of nurses not performing similarly in ways that matter to patients—that is, for example, you may have the same *number* of nursing hours per patient day in various units, but the *quality* of the patient interactions is variable. Perhaps the nurses are trained or oriented differently, or use different protocols for patient education and patient/family support in various units.

Conversely, a strong correlation should be a call to action to address staffing issues, because they appear to have an impact on patient satisfaction. If the relationship is clear and powerful, then it is important (for your own organization, as well as for JCAHO compliance) to show that you will use these findings to improve operations.

Bear in mind that the level of patient satisfaction is almost certainly not driven by a single HR characteristic. There may be an interaction of several variables that contribute to patient outcomes. For example, after you have worked with your data for a period of time, you may want to increase the sophistication of your analysis. Consider these ideas:

1. Does the *tenure* of your nurses contribute to satisfaction? Is it the case that units with lower turnover and longer employment histories within your hospital seem able to deliver higher levels of satisfaction? To explore this, you would repeat all of the steps outlined in this book but use either turnover or employment tenure as your HR measure.

2. Does the *mix* of your staff contribute to satisfaction? Your hypothesis may be that units with a higher proportion of registered nurses will have higher levels of patient satisfaction. In this case, your HR measure would be the percentage of RNs to total nursing personnel per unit.

Note that these drill-down or more sophisticated analyses should also take into account the factor you have already established—that overall nursing hours per patient day is a powerful factor. There are two ways to address this, depending on how your organization has used the results of your staffing effectiveness analysis.

First, perhaps your hospital has integrated the staffing effectiveness data into operations and is now able to ensure that all patient units are staffed at the appropriate level of nursing hours per patient day. In this case, you would have *no* remaining variability in "nursing hours per patient day," since all clinically similar units would have attained the same staffing pattern. The *r* would drop to near zero, since there is no variation to explain any more. This would be a signal that it is time to explore a new variable, such as those sketched above.

Second, perhaps you have not yet been able to bring all units to a consistent staffing pattern, but you still want to explore additional levels of analysis. While beyond the scope of most hospitals' ambitions at this point and beyond the scope of this book, the strategy you will want to pursue is a multifactorial analysis. This will account for the nursing hours per patient day and address another variable, such as staff turnover, sequentially. For additional reading suggestions in stepwise multiple logistic regression and multifactorial analysis, see Kleinbaum, D. G., and Kupper, L. L. *Applied Regression Analysis and Other Multivariable Methods,* Duxbury Press, Boston, MA, 1978.

This degree of complex statistical analysis is not required for JCAHO compliance.

Section III: Step-by-Step Guide to Meeting the Staffing Effectiveness Standards

Benchmarking and Comparisons

Benchmarking is an important tool for any organization, both because the JCAHO's PI standards require it and because most of us want to ensure that we are holding ourselves to an appropriately high standard. If we don't make these aggressive comparisons ourselves, the payer and government communities will most certainly make them for us.

Comparative data for selected, evidence-based patient care practices and outcomes are available through the federal Quality Improvement Organizations (formerly known as Peer Review Organizations), the JCAHO's ORYX database (managed by intermediary vendors—check with yours), and many other public and private sources, including hospital associations; medical specialty societies; employer and insurer coalitions; and private companies, such as Solucient. The federal government will publish selected process measures by 2004 as part of the national heath care quality report.

Staffing benchmarks are also available, primarily in research literature as cited previously, and are gradually being pulled into proposed and/or adopted state-level legislation mandating defined staffing levels. Proposals at the federal level also rely on this research, and new studies and surveys are steadily appearing, attempting to link staffing levels to specific complications, clinical outcomes, and even mortality.

Most of these staffing benchmarks, however, are difficult to relate to a specific hospital's staffing effectiveness program. Because these studies are typically developed on large databases or are meta-analyses of other studies, it is almost impossible to bring back a number or a formula or relationship that you can rely upon to help you establish the "right" staffing for a specific outcome. Published studies lack important details about the patient populations, staffing models, and other variables, which make all the difference when you attempt to apply their insight to a particular unit or population in your own hospital. "The devil can be in the details," indeed.

Similarly, there are benchmarks for patient satisfaction among most of the major vendors. If you do use a vendor-supported system, you can probably obtain some comparable data to indicate how your survey results compare to other hospitals' results. However, there are no national standards or published studies that definitively link patient satisfaction to staffing levels.

Benchmarking and Comparisons (cont.)

This is not a surprise. Clearly, there are going to be many complex intervening variables, including: staffing mix and competence; patient population and delivery model; physical facility; region; and competitive environment. If you are able to develop a comparable data set with a small number of other hospitals—perhaps within your corporate system or within other hospitals who use the same satisfaction survey vendor—you may be able to define a meaningful benchmarking process that would truly shed new light on this complex dynamic.

Such a benchmarking process can entail a significant amount of work, since it requires careful data collection to ensure comparability. You may all collect patient satisfaction data on the same survey, but do you

- Have comparable response rates?

- Use similar patient care processes, or understand the differences? (Is one an academic medical center, the other a community hospital?)

- Have similar patient populations? (If one hospital has a huge obstetrics population and another a huge geriatrics population, for example, you would expect differences.)

- Measure the same types of staff (direct, indirect) in your HR variable?

- Measure the same staffing—paid hours per patient day, or FTEs per bed, or whatever you have agreed on?

- Include or exclude agency staff in the same way?

- Average the HR data per day, week, month or quarter in the same algorithm?

Of course, the real value in benchmarking is in the very process of exploring the data and comparing how different organizations approach problem solving and data management. Once you have the data, the most creative work then is using the findings to spur effective and efficient improvement using the best insights you have been able to glean from the others in your shared process.

SECTION III: STEP-BY-STEP GUIDE TO MEETING THE STAFFING EFFECTIVENESS STANDARDS

Summarizing the results

When you take your data back to the oversight or quality committee, you will need to present the information in a way that is compelling and meaningful. The raw data are overwhelming and dense, and your careful analysis has resulted in a concise picture of patterns, which suggest possible action. The challenge now is to return to the committee with a strong presentation.

Begin with the original hypothesis: *"We think that patient satisfaction with nursing is probably related to the number of paid nursing hours per inpatient day."* You will now "build a case" to present to the group and trigger appropriate action.

Presentation note:

- One way of stating a hypothesis is that there is no relationship between the two indicators. This is known as the null hypothesis—no relationship. Having selected nursing hours per patient day (HR) and patient satisfaction clinical as our indicators, our *null* hypothesis would be that differences in nursing hours per patient day are not related to differences in patient satisfaction. If your *r* value is very near zero, you will not be able to reject the null hypothesis.

  This is a typical approach in scientific research, and you may find this to be a preferable approach, if the committee is composed of physicians and others accustomed to this style of developing a hypothesis. More commonly however, management and medical leaders dealing with quality data, they will expect the hypothesis to be articulated in a positive direction, as described above: *"We think that patient satisfaction with nursing is probably related to the number of paid nursing hours per inpatient day."* Or, perhaps, *"We will investigate whether there is a relationship between patient satisfaction and paid nursing hours per inpatient day."*

- If you do assert a hypothesis that the two indicators are related, you will need to indicate the level of significance of the relationship, as well as your probability of error of rejecting the null hypothesis. "Significance" means simply your degree of certainty. If your results are

  $$r^2 = 0.45, p < 0.01$$

  then this means that there is a fairly strong, consistent relationship between the two indicators, and the probability that the result is due to chance is less than 1.0 in 100.

  You can generate *p* values when you use the regression function in Excel.

Opportunities for further investigation

Under most circumstances, there is opportunity for further investigation. If you show a correlation, the committee will want to explore actions needed, but it should also consider the possibility of exploring other factors.

- The absence of a correlation is not the end of the search for relationships. It may tell you, however, that you need to search elsewhere. If a small *r* leads you to accept the null hypothesis that your two indicators are *not* related, you will want to examine other causes or variables that may be contributing to your clinical indicators. For example, as suggested above, you may need to examine other factors (besides nurse staffing per patient day) contributing to patient satisfaction levels.

  Thus, the operational implications would include looking for other opportunities and changing practice/behavior where applicable. Keep in mind that it is unlikely that that there will ever be a single absolute factor driving satisfaction levels.

When there is a strong correlation between HR and clinical indicators, you must turn to operational analysis to determine how to optimize staffing and patient outcomes, perhaps through PI mechanisms already in place at your hospital. We'll talk more about action steps in the "What to do next?" section at the end of this book.

Presenting your data

Although you have probably spent months—or years—designing studies and entering data into a spreadsheet or other data collection tool, few people besides you and your work group will actually look at your data. The power of data lies in its presentation, and, although the spreadsheet leads you to it, presentation is more of a key than a doorway.

For most audiences, you will use the information in your data collection tool (in our case, an Excel spreadsheet) to create a graphic presentation of your data. Yes, there is a measure of redundancy in presenting the spreadsheet data in one or many graphics, but the value lies in visualization—"a picture is worth a thousand words." When you are summarizing large amounts of data, a graphic presentation may draw attention to significant features that are difficult to observe in a column of numbers (as they appear in a spreadsheet).

What type of graphic presentation you choose depends a lot on your audience. Who will look at your data? Key audiences include your hospital's leadership (this is required by the JCAHO), PI/QI

Section III: Step-by-Step Guide to Meeting the Staffing Effectiveness Standards

committees, decision-making boards, perhaps state regulatory bodies, and, of course, the JCAHO survey team itself. It is unlikely that you will print out and distribute your spreadsheet to any of the above audiences. They do not need that level of detail.

If you present your data to a JCAHO surveyor, it is unlikely that he or she will want the detail found in your spreadsheet (other than as proof of documentation). The surveyor will want to look at your analysis for any trends. For example, you may have demonstrated that patient satisfaction is strongest in areas with a given level of staffing. Did the committee review and evaluate this relationship with staffing? What's your next step?

What type of graphic presentation you choose may also depend on what you are trying to show. For example, if you are trying to change staff behavior by showing the staff on Unit 1 that your data shows a correlation between nursing hours and patient satisfaction for that unit, your presentation would center around Unit 1—not Unit 2, Unit 3, or all the units combined.

Based on your audience and the point you wish to convey, you may use many types of graphs to present your data. For the purpose of this book, we'll be looking at three of the most common graphs: bar charts, x-y plots, and run charts (we discussed run charts in the Establishing control limits on page 65).

Regardless of the graphs you choose, they should meet the following requirements:

- Your graphs should show data without misrepresenting or distorting it. For example, basing your presentation on a small number of data points—typically anything fewer than 15–30—would be a misrepresentation.

- Your graphs should not sidetrack the audience, who should be thinking about what the data shows, not about how you created the chart. You will want to save valuable committee member time by avoiding unnecessary questions about the construction of the graphs due to omission of titles, labels, scales, etc.

- Your graphs should encourage comparison of different data pieces.

- Your choice of graphs will probably depend on your personal comfort with the data underlying the graphs and graphic styles, as well as the prevailing conventions at your organization.

Section III: Step-by-Step Guide to Meeting the Staffing Effectiveness Standards

Our sample charts show the type of information you may want to share with a variety of audiences, including departmental and board quality committees. Before introducing your graph illustrating the staffing effectiveness relationship you are studying, it is essential to provide clear definitions of every measure. Thus, when you introduce the graphic presentation, everyone in your audience will be able to focus on results instead of definitional details.

In some circumstances, you will want to review and present comparative data. It may take one of the following forms:

- Baseline or trends in measures. What is the level of performance before introducing a change in practice? What sort of history of performance is there?

- External comparison, if available. How are other hospitals performing with staffing effectiveness (HR and clinical indicator relationships)?

You will want to explain what the *desired performance* should be. If you already have organizational goals for patient satisfaction, this target will be defined for you. If there are discrepancies between the desired and actual performances in your hospital, you will be offering assistance by using staffing effectiveness data to help explain how to close the gap.

As you look at our sample graphs, it is important to remember that we are using the graphs to look at many different factors—not only the relationship between the indicators. Bar charts, for example, do not allow you to graph both measures (patient satisfaction and nursing hours per patient day) within the same graph, so we will be looking at these types of graphs for clues about our data. Bar charts are more for our own use (i.e. the use of the data collection team) because they do not convey the results of the <u>relationship.</u> Thus, as we demonstrate different types of graphs, do not look immediately for the relationship/correlation. In many of the graphs, we will only be exploring and looking for insight into our data.

Section III: Step-by-Step Guide to Meeting the Staffing Effectiveness Standards

Presenting to the JCAHO

As we mentioned earlier, it is unlikely that your surveyor will want to view a printout of your entire spreadsheet, other than as documentation that you have, in fact, been collecting data. So, what should you show them?

Because the JCAHO's standards are nonprescriptive about what data you should collect, how you should analyze it, and what you should do with your results, the key to meeting this standard is **knowledge.** You need to be able to prove, through leadership and staff interviews, that staffing effectiveness is an area of focus at your hospital. This means that

- leaders are aware of the concept of staffing effectiveness
- leaders know what measures you are tracking, and, in general terms, what the measures reveal
- leaders can discuss actions taken, or under consideration, as a result of the analysis and discussion that has occurred

The relevant leaders will be at least those in the areas whose staff are included in the analysis (e.g., nursing, housekeeping, dietary, etc.), depending on what decisions you made in defining your indicators.

The key activity specified by the JCAHO in its staffing effectiveness standards is the **correlation of measures**—that is, examining relationships between HR and clinical indicators—and **action based on the results.** The only way to approach this task effectively is to select indicators, gather data, analyze the data, and interpret the results—the steps you are already taking for all of your PI projects—as suggested above. From these data, the JCAHO will look for results that you should be paying attention to, such as trends, and will interview leaders to assess their awareness and action plans based on the results.

Monitoring your results will close the loop in your process toward meeting the JCAHO's staffing effectiveness standard and improving patient satisfaction within your hospital. You will need to track patient satisfaction and clinical outcomes related to HR indicators from the beginning of any patient satisfaction improvement initiative to ensure that your interventions are producing the desired and planned results.

SECTION III: STEP-BY-STEP GUIDE TO MEETING THE STAFFING EFFECTIVENESS STANDARDS

Exploring the data: Graphic and statistical processes

Bar chart

A bar chart is a distribution of measure values (nursing hours) over time (i.e., months—a common dimension of the measure).

The data you use in your bar chart depends on your audience and what you want to highlight within your graph. For example, if you want to illustrate that staffing levels are similar across your patient care units, you may present a bar chart showing similar nursing hours for similar types of patient care units—that is, with the same number of beds, similar types of patients, etc. If you want to illustrate differences, you may use the bar chart to show very different numbers of nursing hours in patient care units of different sizes providing care to very different types of patients.

> **Creating Charts in Excel**
>
> To create a chart within your Excel spreadsheet:
>
> 1. Highlight the data within your spreadsheet that you would like to include in your chart.
>
> 2. Select "Insert" from the toolbar at the top of your screen.
>
> 3. Select "Chart" from the drop-down menu that appears.
>
> 4. You will then be taken through a "Chart Wizard," the step-by-step process of selecting chart type and data source, titling your chart and x-y axis, etc.

Some general features to note (either in construction or interpretation) when using a bar chart include the following:

- What gets to be the x-axis vs. the y-axis? For bar charts, the horizontal axis (x-axis) is made up of categories (e.g., units of time such as months), while the vertical axis (y-axis) is based on values taken on by the categories (e.g., nursing hours in the study month).

- Horizontal bars vs. vertical bars. The bars in a bar chart may be positioned horizontally or vertically. Horizontal bars allow you to display long category labels. The defaults in Excel chart production also allow more space for labels along the vertical axis. Long labels associated with the x-axis may be truncated, placed at angles, broken into letter groups in multiple rows, etc.

Section III: Step-by-Step Guide to Meeting the Staffing Effectiveness Standards

- Labels

    - **Title**—Your title should include sufficient information about your data so that the graph's contents are clear when separated from other documentation. You will want to include the study period, the measures being presented, and possibly the topic of data being presented.

    - **Axis titles**—If you choose to present nursing hours by months, a horizontal axis title for the bar chart is probably not necessary since the axis labels (month "names") make the axis title self-explanatory. If you were to include an axis title, however, it would be something like "activity period." You would want to title the horizontal axis if the measure represented is not obvious by the axis labels.

    - **Legend**—Legends should be used to identify multiple data sets. If you chose to present two patient care units of data for each month, the bar chart would have two bars for each month. The legend would document the locations (e.g., patient care unit) associated with each of the pairs of bars.

    - **Footnotes**—Information about the data or the presentation that is not contained in the chart or axis titles may be reserved for footnotes. You may want to place warnings, such as a confidentiality notice on the presentation, in your footnotes to protect your data from inappropriate uses. It is also extremely important to include the source of the data, the analyst preparing the chart, the date of development, and possibly the name of the file.

    - **Data labels**—Data labels are sometimes included on bar charts to clarify the values represented by the height of the bars. Not all values are convenient to present. They're not always necessary either if the values are clear from the vertical axis. When the numbers are reasonably short, their presence can make the variation in the distribution clearer.

Bar charts are sometimes used to present chronological data that illustrate trends. Keep in mind that bars do not account for the uneven intervals of time that you may have in your data. Trend lines (discussed later) are another way of presenting chronological data.

To demonstrate the use of bar charts in a presentation, we've created a bar chart for each of the columns of our hypothetical hospital's spreadsheet. Some of these bar charts may be important to the staffing effectiveness initiative team, while others simply help you, the data collector, visualize the data for yourself.

SECTION III: STEP-BY-STEP GUIDE TO MEETING THE STAFFING EFFECTIVENESS STANDARDS

Let's look at our hypothetical data again.

Bar charts have been created from columns B–F in the Excel spreadsheet. These are presented in groups related to the type of data below. The first three bar charts are for the data you entered for nursing hours (Chart 11), patient satisfaction scores (Chart 12), and patient days (Chart 13) by month.

The bar chart below illustrates the distribution of monthly nursing hours. This chart is derived from the data in Column B, rows 3-20, of the Excel spreadsheet. On the horizontal axis (x-axis), the months are identified. The number of nursing hours associated with them are represented by the height of the bars.

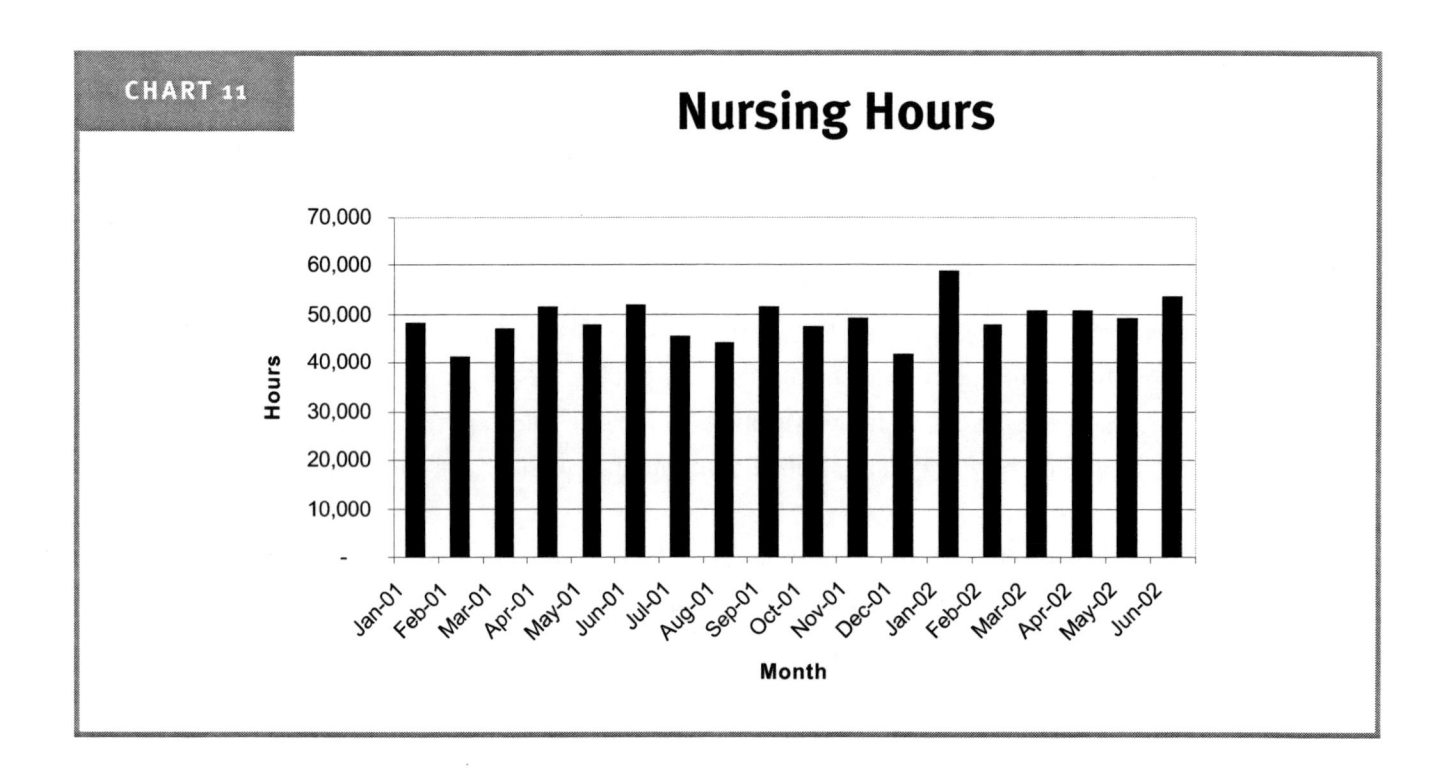

CHART 11

Nursing Hours

108 INCREASING PATIENT SATISFACTION WITH STATISTICAL CORRELATION

SECTION III: STEP-BY-STEP GUIDE TO MEETING THE STAFFING EFFECTIVENESS STANDARDS

While nursing hours seem to vary across the months, we don't have enough information to know whether the variations are appropriate, in light of the census and other factors.

Chart 12 illustrates the distribution of patient satisfaction scores by month. This chart is derived from the data in Column E, rows 3-20, of our Excel spreadsheet. On the horizontal axis, the calendar months are identified. Patient satisfaction levels are represented by the height of the bars and are labeled on the vertical axis. As you can see, there is variability across months. The mean patient satisfaction is displayed by the black line that appears horizontally across the middle of the chart.

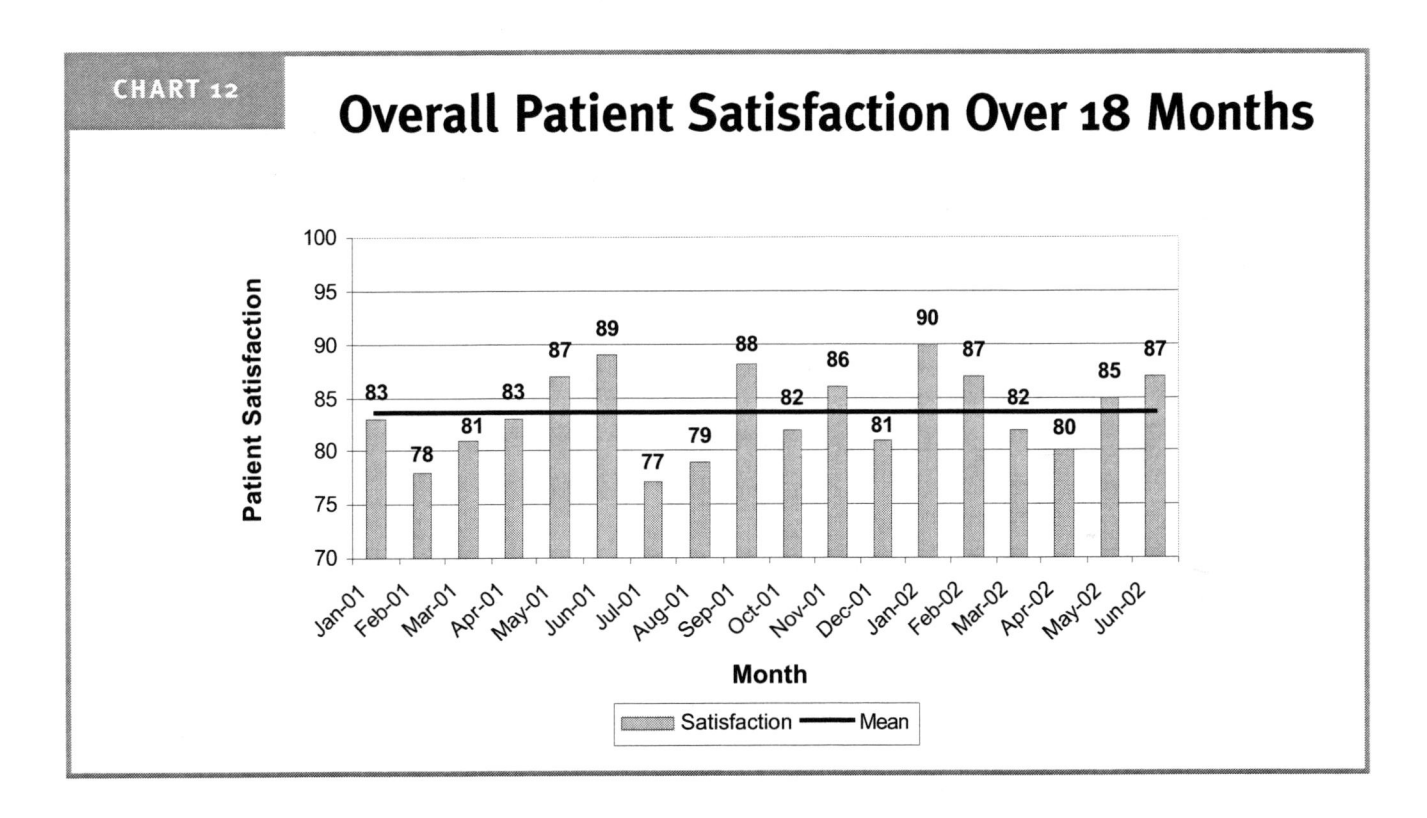

CHART 12

Overall Patient Satisfaction Over 18 Months

Month	Satisfaction
Jan-01	83
Feb-01	78
Mar-01	81
Apr-01	83
May-01	87
Jun-01	89
Jul-01	77
Aug-01	79
Sep-01	88
Oct-01	82
Nov-01	86
Dec-01	81
Jan-02	90
Feb-02	87
Mar-02	82
Apr-02	80
May-02	85
Jun-02	87

You can draw several conclusions from this chart: Satisfaction appears to be variable, and there is no obvious trend as far as seasons of the year, or overall change during the period. We don't know what the census was in these study periods or the staffing needed to take care of the number of patients in the hospital. We also have not examined the mix of patients (medical, surgical, OB) or clinical acuity. So, we will need other information to try to understand these fluctuations.

INCREASING PATIENT SATISFACTION WITH STATISTICAL CORRELATION

SECTION III: STEP-BY-STEP GUIDE TO MEETING THE STAFFING EFFECTIVENESS STANDARDS

Chart 13 illustrates the distribution of patient days by calendar month. This chart is derived from the data in Column C, rows 3-20, of the Excel spreadsheet. On the horizontal axis, the months are identified. The number of patient days associated with them are represented by the height of the bars and are labeled on the vertical axis. As you can see, there is variability across time.

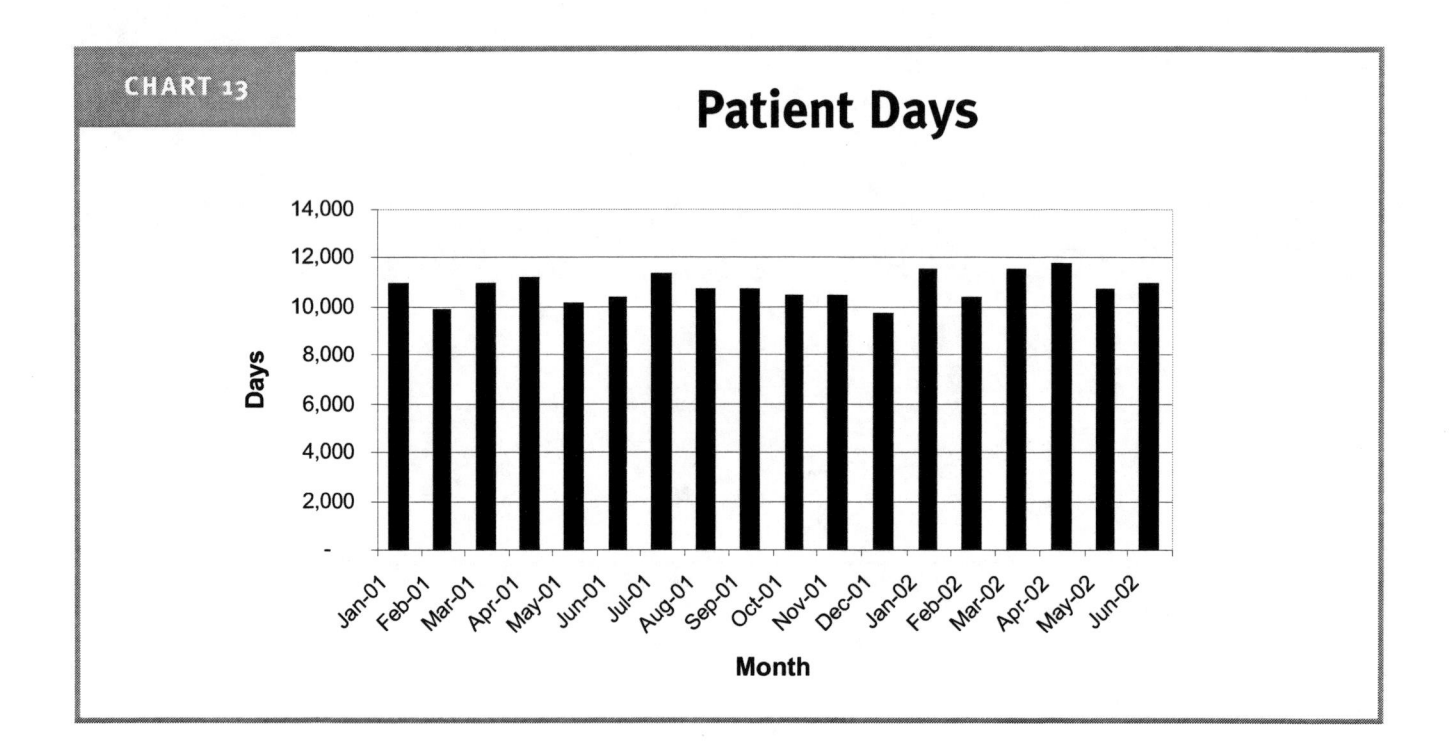

CHART 13

Patient Days

The conclusion you can draw from this chart is that there is some variability in the number of patient days during the months of the study period. We don't know, however, what significance this may have for patient satisfaction.

SECTION III: STEP-BY-STEP GUIDE TO MEETING THE STAFFING EFFECTIVENESS STANDARDS

Creating bar charts for measures based on two other measures

The second group of bar charts illustrates columns of data derived from two other measures. These measures appear in columns D and F. These charts are Chart 14 and Chart 15.

In Chart 14, you can see that nursing hours per patient day by month were fairly uniform across the study period, although there may be a slight increasing trend. From this bar chart, you do not know what types of patients' needs were being filled, or which resulted in patient satisfaction.

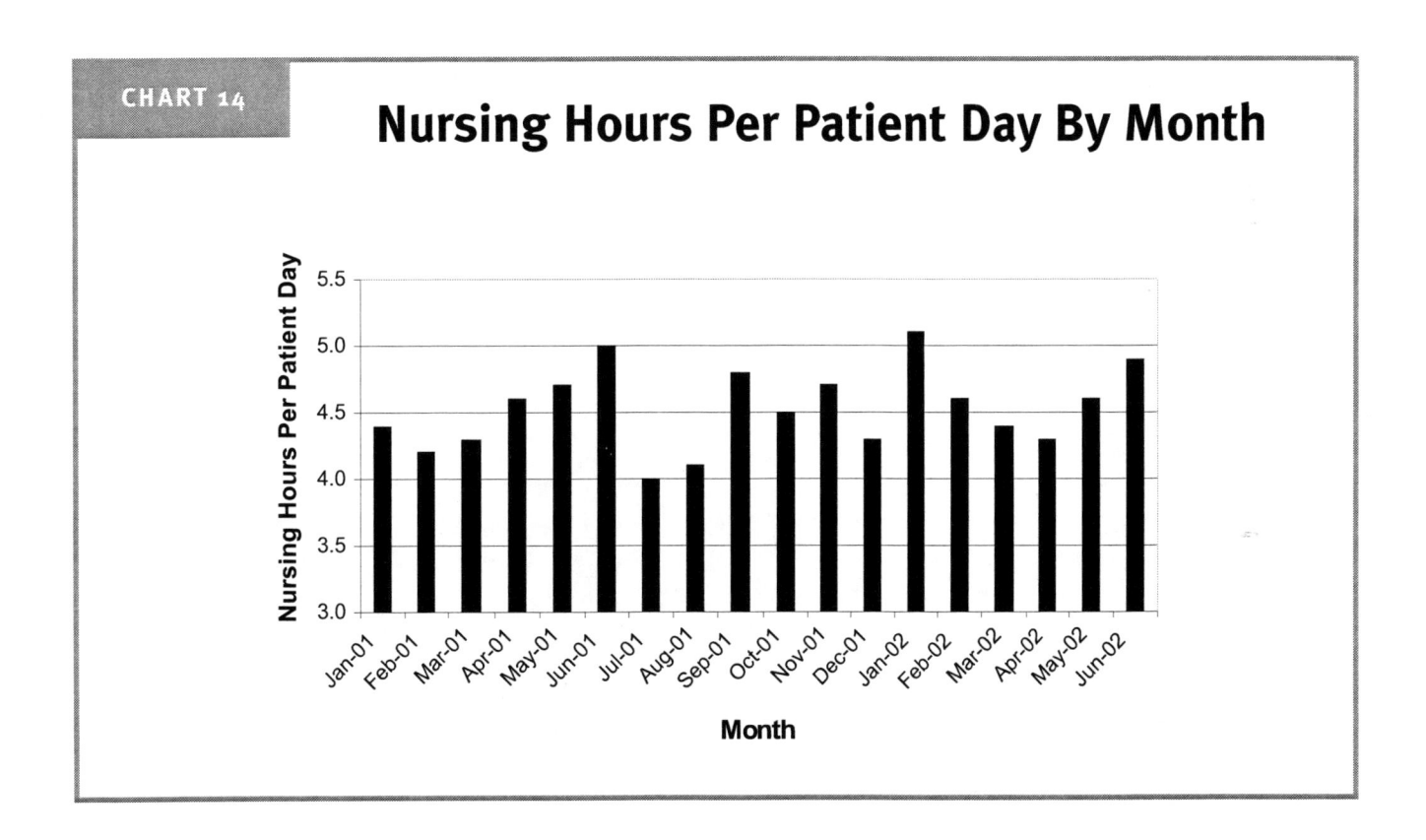

CHART 14: Nursing Hours Per Patient Day By Month

Section III: Step-by-Step Guide to Meeting the Staffing Effectiveness Standards

Chart 15 illustrates the distribution of the monthly ratio of patient satisfaction scores to nursing hours per patient day.

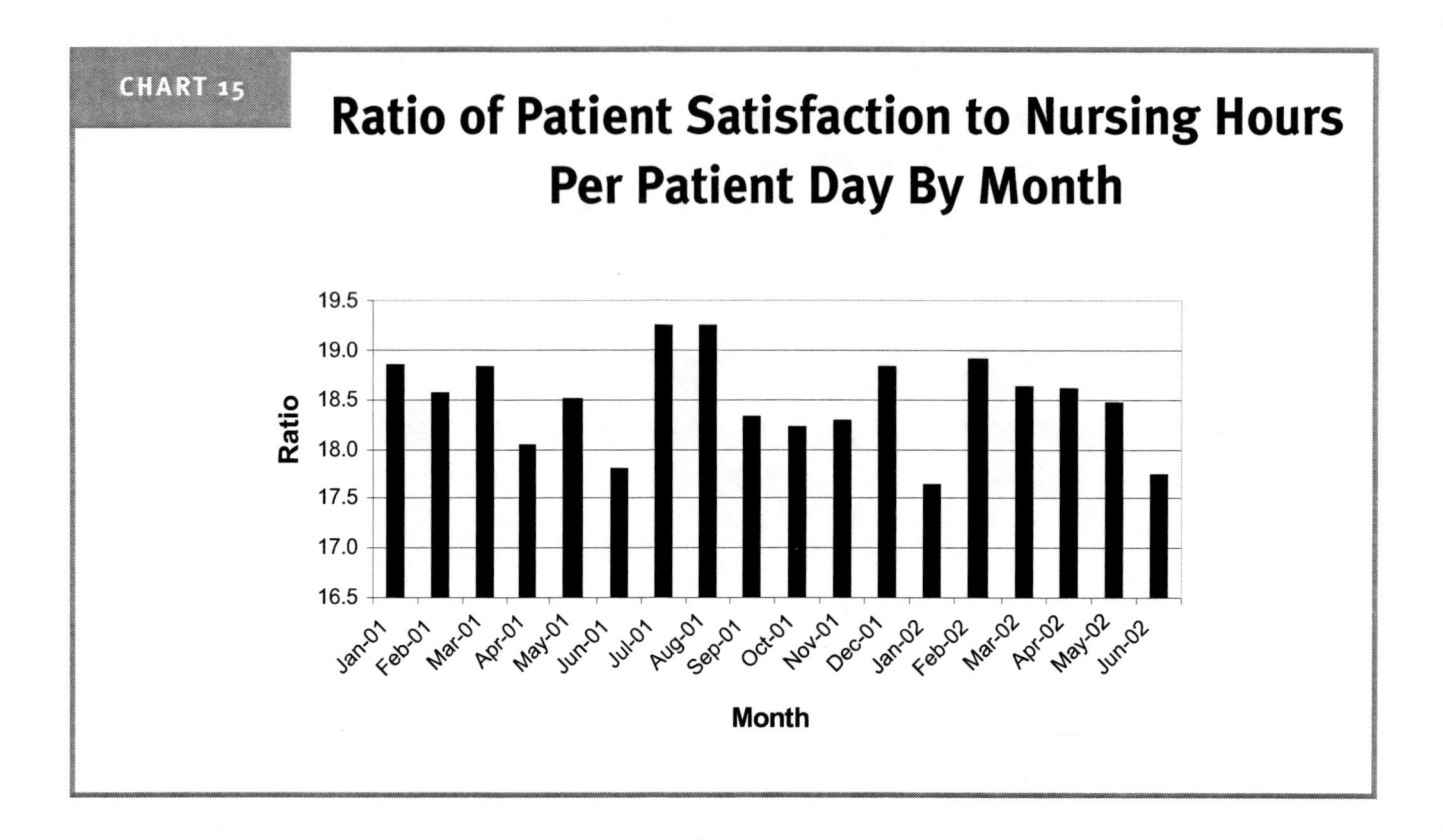

CHART 15

Ratio of Patient Satisfaction to Nursing Hours Per Patient Day By Month

As you can see, there appear to be fluctuations in the ratio of patient satisfaction scores to nursing hours per patient day over time, although we cannot be sure why, or whether these changes are statistically significant, at this point. The next step is to compare this data with the nursing hours data to determine what type of correlations and conclusions you can draw concerning staffing's influencing patient satisfaction with nursing care. To do this, we will introduce the concept of an x-y plot or a scattergram—*"scatterplot."*

Section III: Step-by-Step Guide to Meeting the Staffing Effectiveness Standards

x-y plots—One measure vs. another

Plotting one measure against another is the object of x-y plots. These plots will incorporate the inferential statistics described above, specifically the r and the r^2. The significance of x-y plots is that they address relationships between staffing effectiveness measures, which is the essence of the JCAHO's staffing effectiveness standards. **Also, x-y plots will show you definitely whether a relationship exists.**

We began looking at x-y plots in "Analyzing Your Data." Let's look at another x-y plot based on our hypothetical hospital's data.

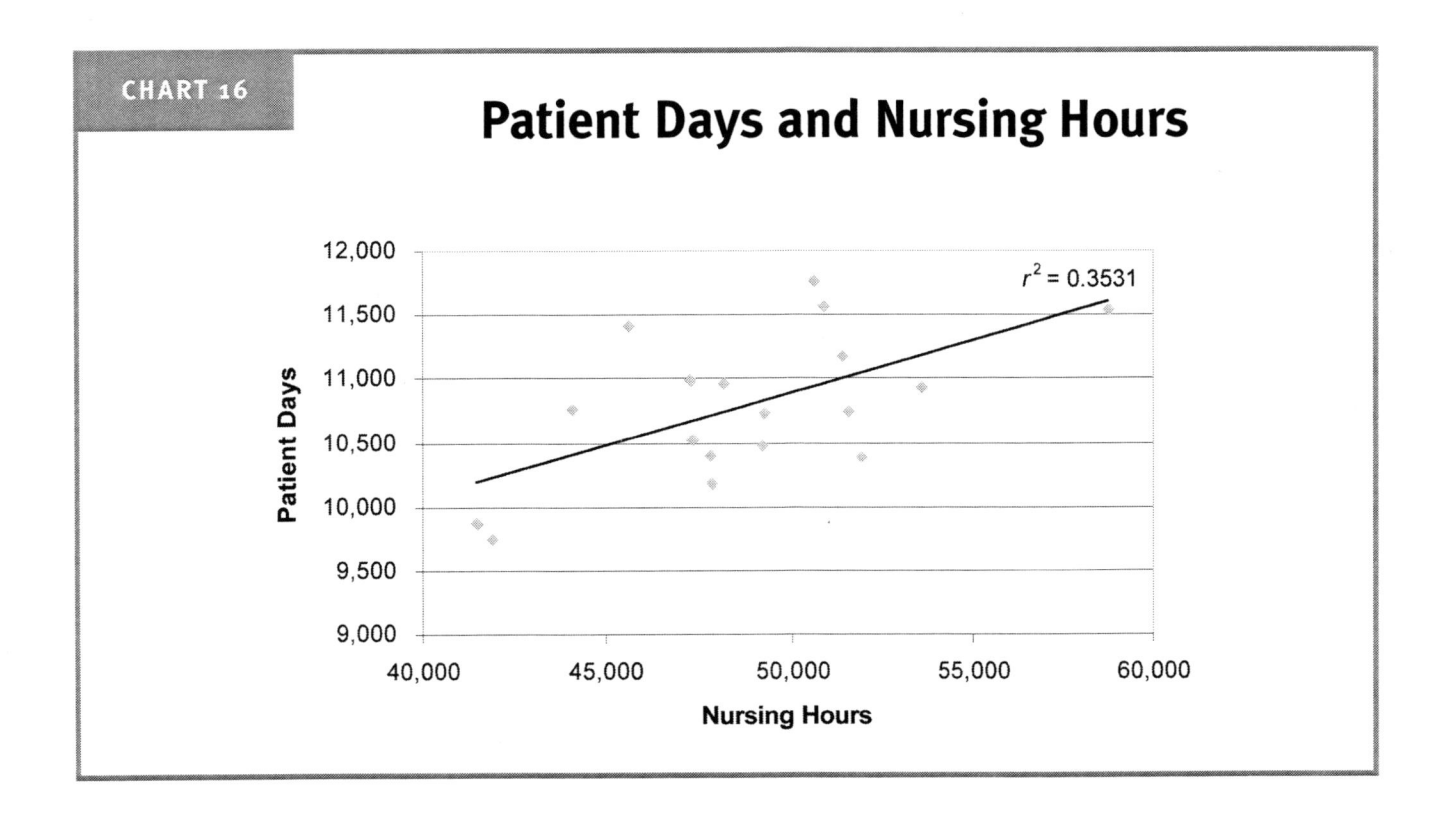

CHART 16

Patient Days and Nursing Hours

$r^2 = 0.3531$

(x-axis: Nursing Hours, 40,000 to 60,000; y-axis: Patient Days, 9,000 to 12,000)

When plotting one measure against another, the "cause" measure is generally associated with the horizontal axis, while the "effect" measure is associated with the vertical axis. For example, in Chart 16, monthly patient days (which translate into demand for nursing care) might be construed as the "cause" for a certain level of staffing (which translates into monthly nursing hours), the "effect." A trend line of the relationship between nursing hours and patient days has been added to the x-y plot.

Increasing Patient Satisfaction With Statistical Correlation

Section III: Step-by-Step Guide to Meeting the Staffing Effectiveness Standards

What does the information in the Chart 16 reveal? First, that there is clearly a relationship, as you would expect. In general the hospital would staff according to patient volume. The r^2 value of 0.35 is equivalent to the *r* value of approximately 0.6. This is a strong relationship and one that should not be surprising. This clearly reflects a management philosophy that flexes staffing to patient volume.

The relationship is not a perfect 1.0, however, for a number of reasons. First, we don't increase staffing by a fraction for each new patient; we adjust to overall ratios and averages. (This is known as a "step function" in cost accounting: We don't typically add one-tenth of a nurse, if two more patients than we expected are admitted on a given day to a 20-bed unit. If the unit begins to see a higher census of three more patients consistently, however, we might consider increasing staffing by a part-time person.) Furthermore, some staffing changes require lead-time to recruit, hire, orient, and train new people. And over time, there will be other factors in our staffing data, such as vacations, personal leave, etc., that may add a little "noise" to the data.

Note the scales on the horizontal and vertical axes. They do not begin with zero. The scales are based on the range of values for monthly patient days and monthly nursing hours. So, the vertical axis begins at 9,000 days, and the horizontal axis begins at 40,000 nursing hours. The x-y plot could be presented with zero as the beginning of both axes, but this is not necessary, since the ranges of values are not near zero. Always examine the scale of a chart before drawing conclusions about trends and patterns that appear as the data are presented. Depending on the scale, a trend or pattern may appear drastically exaggerated or understated, which might result in your drawing incorrect conclusions about your data.

SECTION III: STEP-BY-STEP GUIDE TO MEETING THE STAFFING EFFECTIVENESS STANDARDS

In Chart 17, monthly patient satisfaction scores are plotted against monthly patient days. Monthly patient days (which translate into how "busy" the hospital is) might be construed as the "cause" for a certain level of satisfaction, the "effect." Thus, this time, the horizontal axis is monthly patient days, and the vertical axis is monthly patient satisfaction. A trend line of the relationship between monthly patient satisfaction and monthly patient days has been added to the x-y plot.

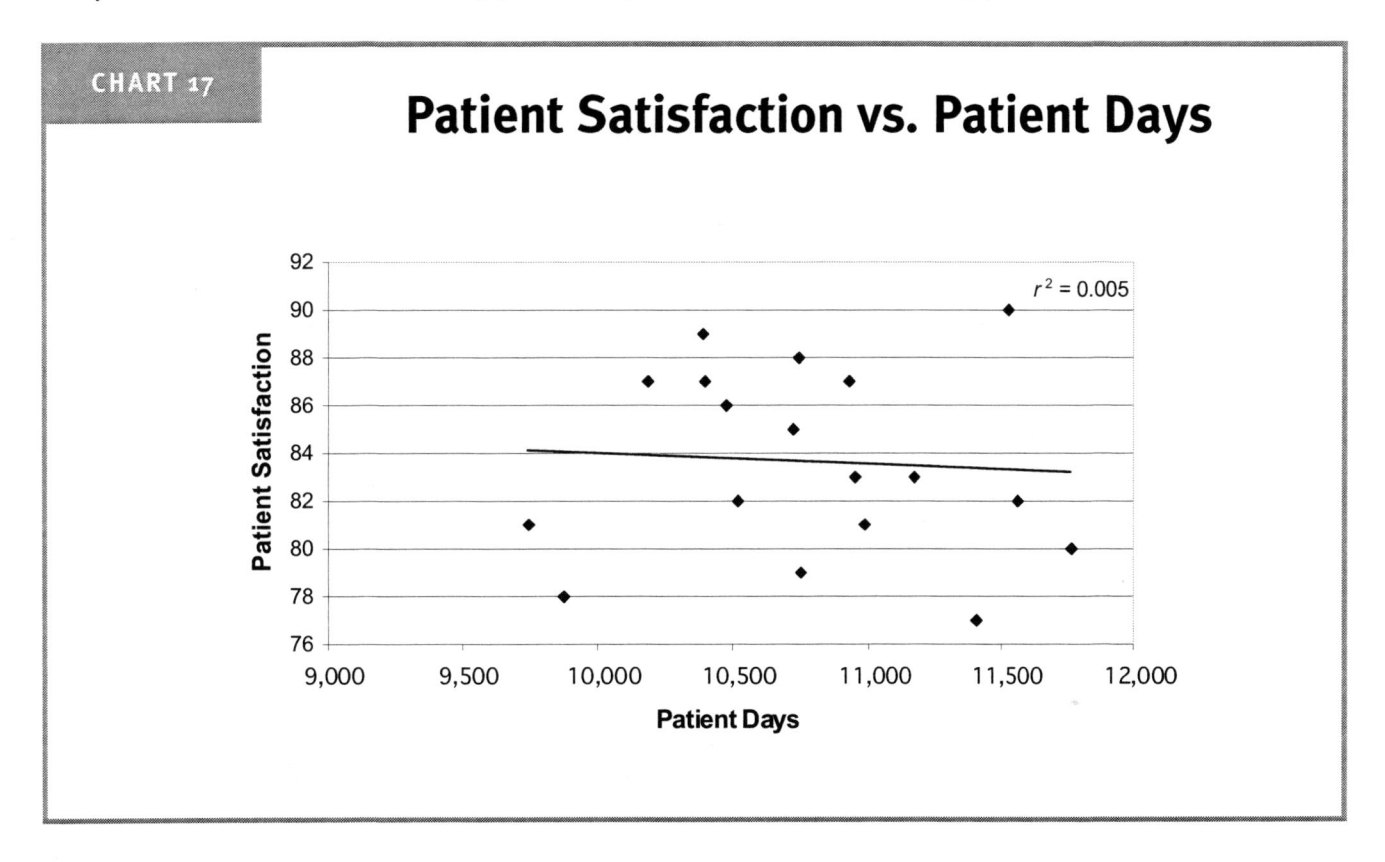

CHART 17

Patient Satisfaction vs. Patient Days

$r^2 = 0.005$

What does the information in this plot reveal? There is clearly no relationship at all between patient satisfaction and total patient days. If we hypothesized that being more "busy" would affect patient satisfaction, this plot would show us that this is *not* the case at all. Neither more nor fewer patient days is predictably associated with any particular level of patient satisfaction. The r^2 value of .005 is vanishingly small.

INCREASING PATIENT SATISFACTION WITH STATISTICAL CORRELATION

SECTION III: STEP-BY-STEP GUIDE TO MEETING THE STAFFING EFFECTIVENESS STANDARDS

The final chart, monthly nursing hours per patient day (which translates into demand for nursing care), might be construed as the "cause" for monthly patient satisfaction level, the "effect." **Chart 18 answers our ultimate question: Is there a relationship between nursing hours per patient day and patient satisfaction?**

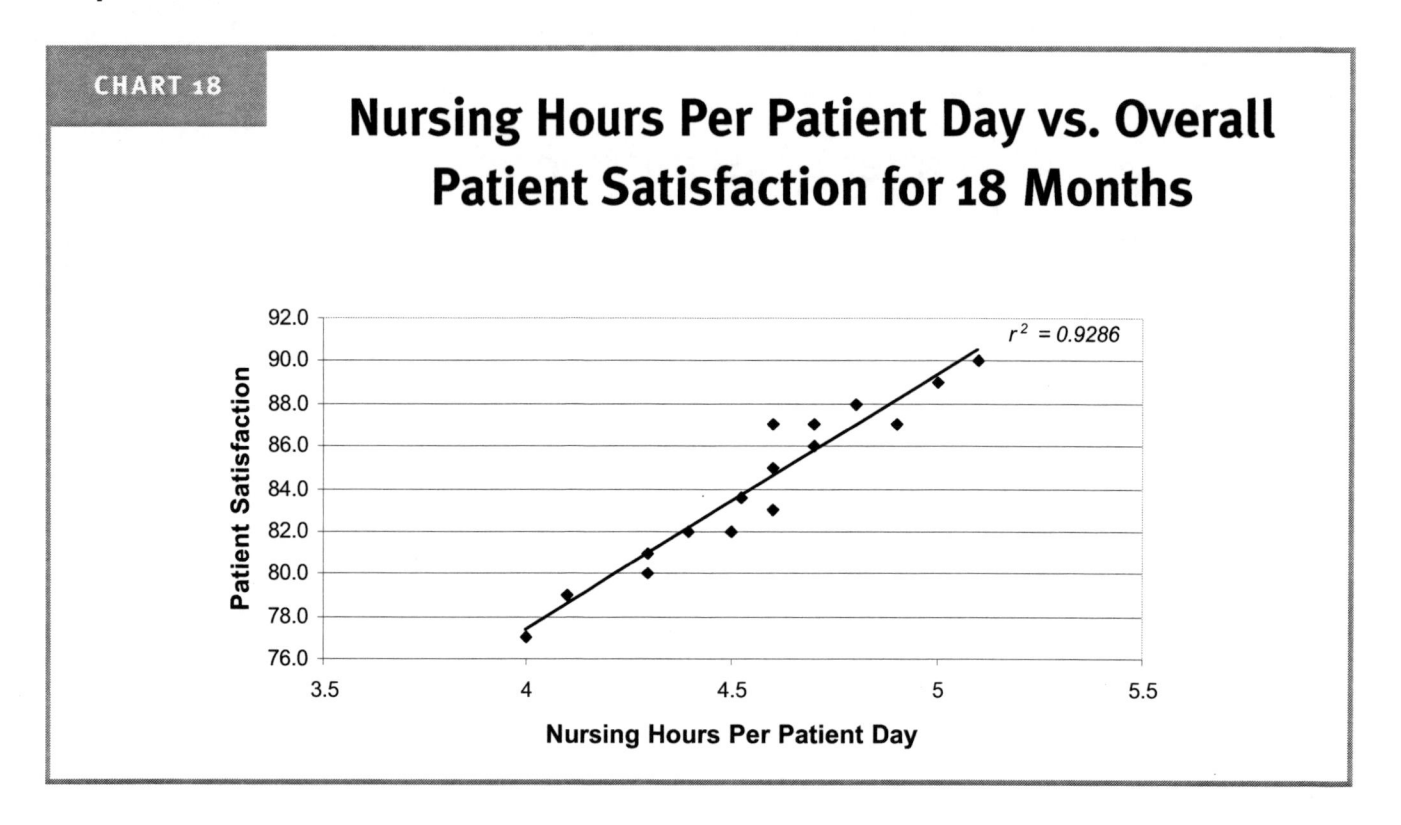

CHART 18

Nursing Hours Per Patient Day vs. Overall Patient Satisfaction for 18 Months

$r^2 = 0.9286$

What does the information in the above chart reveal? **There is an obvious and powerful relationship between patient satisfaction on the y-axis and nursing hours per patient day on the x-axis.** The r^2 of 0.93 reflects an underlying correlation exceeding 0.9, an exceptionally strong relationship.

It is important that your oversight committee clearly understands that there is no direct relationship between patient satisfaction and patient days ("busy-ness") or between patient satisfaction and the absolute number of nursing hours (gross staffing levels). The relationship is with the *number of nursing hours available per number of patients in the hospital specifically*.

In fact, you can be even more specific. *If you deliver about 4.5–4.7 hours per patient day of nursing care, you will consistently improve patient satisfaction with nursing care.*

Section III: Step-by-Step Guide to Meeting the Staffing Effectiveness Standards

We will review the implications of this important observation for operational action and improvement in the conclusion.

For full compliance with JCAHO expectations for staffing effectiveness and performance improvement, you will need to ensure that your committee reviews the data and discusses the implications fully.

A working format for presenting a summary to your committee is included in Figure 6. You will want to conduct a full presentation with background, the process to date, and the results. This should include the following:

- Review the basic requirements of the JCAHO's standards.
- Review the charter of the group's and the organization's priorities for improvement of patient satisfaction.
- Revalidate the appropriateness of the measures, the data collection, and manipulation. Ensure that the group clearly understands and endorses the data definitions (e.g. which types of staff were included in the HR measure)
- Reverify the relevance of the measure to overall organizational goals and priorities.
- Examine the data, step by step, to confirm the analysis and ensure that no issues or problems exist that could compromise the validity of the data.
- Draw conclusions as a group, regarding the relationship of nurse staffing to patient satisfaction.
- Discuss recommendations (See below).

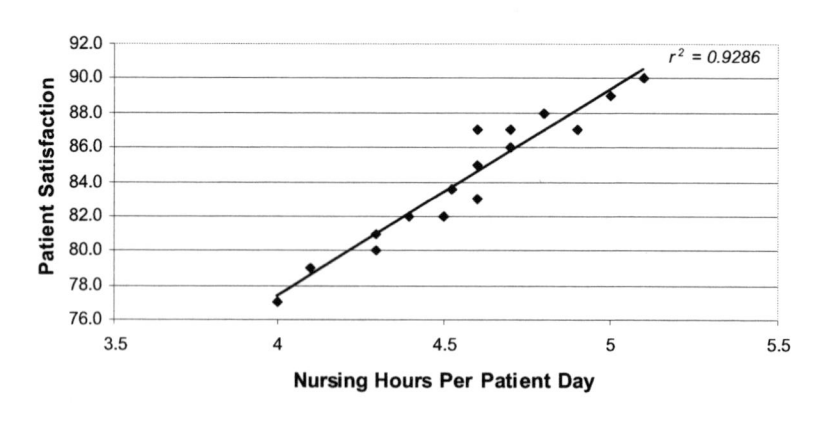

SECTION III: STEP-BY-STEP GUIDE TO MEETING THE STAFFING EFFECTIVENESS STANDARDS

FIGURE 6

Example: Quality Improvement Planning and Monitoring

Example Memorial Hospital

Quality Improvement Planning and Monitoring	Date:

PROCESS: Staffing Effectiveness

Overview, History, Why Important:

Measure: *Patient satisfaction with nursing care*
Executive Leadership Summary: *The following departments have been involved in the evaluation of staffing effectiveness: nursing, finance, human resources, and quality (under the auspices of the Quality Improvement Committee/Staffing Effectiveness Subcommittee).*

A strong correlation was found between patient satisfaction with nursing, and nursing hours per patient day. Recommendations are listed below. Monitoring will continue after intervention to ensure effective action.

The hospital's strategic goal was to improve patient satisfaction at least ___%. Nursing satisfaction is known to be a key driver of overall satisfaction.

Performance Dimensions and Goals:
Staffing Effectiveness Measure Set 1: Hypothesis: Nurse staffing has a relationship to patient satisfaction on the nursing-related survey questions.

Current Period Performance:
Statistical relationship is confirmed.

Nursing Hours Per Patient Day vs. Overall Patient Satisfaction For 18 Months

$r^2 = 0.9286$

INCREASING PATIENT SATISFACTION WITH STATISTICAL CORRELATION

Section III: Step-by-Step Guide to Meeting the Staffing Effectiveness Standards

FIGURE 6

Example: Quality Improvement Planning and Monitoring (cont.)

Trend: Performance Over Time:
Process is stable.

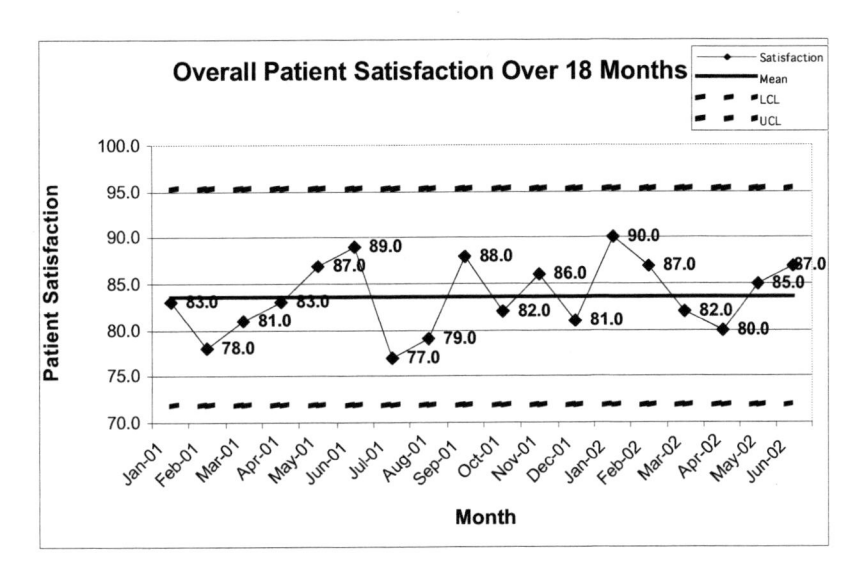

Overall Patient Satisfaction Over 18 Months

Data points (Jan-01 through Jun-02): 83.0, 78.0, 81.0, 83.0, 87.0, 89.0, 77.0, 79.0, 88.0, 82.0, 86.0, 81.0, 90.0, 87.0, 82.0, 80.0, 85.0, 87.0

Legend: Satisfaction, Mean, LCL, UCL

FINDINGS AND CONCLUSIONS

Are the measures linked? What evidence of statistical relationship do you have?
These measures are significantly linked. There is an r^2 of .92 between nursing hours per patient day and patient satisfaction with nursing. There is NO relationship between patient satisfaction and total nursing hours, nor with total patient days.

Is staffing effective to achieve the desired outcome at this time? How do you know?
There is an opportunity to improve patient satisfaction by evaluating staffing ratios in each unit and ensuring that they all meet optimum levels. When variability among units is decreased, overall patient satisfaction will improve.

If not, what are team conclusions about potential areas for improvement?
Team recommends unit-specific analyses in conjunction with budget process, to identify which areas may be under or over staffed.

FIGURE 6: Example: Quality Improvement Planning and Monitoring (cont.)

What additional data, pilot studies, small-scale tests of change, etc. are needed?
Drill down to the unit level. In conjunction with budget discussions, may need to look at specific nursing behaviors on the units with higher staffing to determine whether we can meet patients' needs for excellent nursing care without increasing total FTEs beyond benchmark ratios. Later evaluations may address the impact of staff turnover, use of protocols to give patients adequate discharge information, etc.

STRATEGIES: Recommendations to be implemented/referred for action

Action	By Whom	By When
• *Analyze staffing by unit to identify high and low units* • *Observe and interview staff/patients to assess key behaviors that result in high patient satisfaction* • *Compare target staffing rations to budget and evaluate differences (above/below)* • *Submit updated budget request* • *Short-term: Consider reallocating staff among units depending on census* • *Long-term: Collect additional data to assess other critical factors for patient satisfaction*		

FOLLOW UP

Date:

Review data again

Update on referred recommendations

Report at unit/department meeting

Report to medical director/clinical leadership

Approved: _____

Conclusion
What to Do Next

Conclusion: What to Do Next

Now that we have reviewed how to collect data, where to find it within your organization, and how to display and present it, let's look further at how to use this information for performance improvement. First, keep in mind that measurement helps to assess and evaluate the level of performance needed to determine if improvement actions are necessary.

As you review the process and prepare for your report to management, keep in mind four key components to data analysis:

1. Determine if any patterns exist in the indicators that are under study during the same time period (bar graphs).
2. Evaluate causes of indicator data results (x-y or scatter plots, r and r^2 statistics).
3. Use committee reflection and brainstorming, and consider other sources of data to expand your review of possible causes for variation.
4. Ensure that data are collected and trended over time to confirm and monitor findings and improvements.

What if you find a correlation?

As demonstrated in the hypothetical case in this book, we used patient satisfaction and nursing hours per patient day to determine if there was a correlation between satisfaction and staffing. In our case, we found a powerful correlation between satisfaction and nursing hours per patient day but not between satisfaction and gross nurse staffing or gross patient days.

This is an important insight for management. Simply increasing or decreasing hours of staffing is *not* indicative of satisfaction based on these data. What is necessary is to determine the *right ratio of staff to patient days*. This is something that will drive additional analyses (discussed further below).

Conclusion: What to do Next

By performing this analysis, we have met the intent of the analysis aspect of the JCAHO's staffing effectiveness standards. We selected two indicators, one clinical, one HR; showed rationale for our selection; defined which caregivers are involved; collected and analyzed data; and demonstrated results through graphs to identify potential staffing effectiveness issues.

Does this mean that you are done? No. You have completed the analysis, but you have yet to undertake the *improvement*. We will address this in a moment.

What if *your* data review did *not* reveal a similar outcome—a positive correlation? Then you will have additional steps to take before moving toward the action phase.

As for the sample data from our hypothetical hospital, until we demonstrate a link back to action, we are *not* finished with our staffing effectiveness effort.

Let's consider both paths.

If there is no correlation

If you can't demonstrate through data analysis a relationship between patient satisfaction using falls to staffing, then to meet the JCAHO's standards, your next step would be to present these findings to hospital leadership. If patient satisfaction is indeed an important hospital goal, however, an additional step would be to use PI techniques to investigate other factors related to satisfaction and to repeat this or similar studies to identify factors that *do* affect this outcome.

If you do find a correlation

The first task with the completed correlation analysis is to figure out what it really means in terms of operational action. You have concluded that there is a relationship between staffing and satisfaction—but what is that relationship exactly, and how will you use the information to improve care and satisfaction?

The data prove that you will deliver higher degrees of patient satisfaction with nursing care if the nursing hours per patient day are maintained at an acceptable level (and if other factors are kept constant, such as staff orientation, training, standards of practice, etc.).

Note that we excluded ICUs from our analysis in this study since we did not have patient satisfaction data for those units. It is critically important, of course, to keep sight of these important decisions concerning data when you are crafting action plans. Otherwise, you might inappropriately try to apply a staffing effectiveness insight developed on the basis of med/surg unit analysis to areas with very different dynamics (e.g., ICUs).

With these data, you can look at your organization's budgets and assess which departments and units can improve their staffing to achieve desired results in patient satisfaction. The data will enable you to begin a discussion of the costs and benefits of staffing changes. Some areas may conceivably be able to reduce staffing and still maintain a range that is acceptable. Others may need to increase staffing to a degree.

The effectiveness of the intervention will depend on your organization's ability to forecast census (patient days) accurately, and to recruit competent staff at a level needed for that census.

A further "drill-down" at this point would be to repeat the entire analysis within specific populations. This would enable you to determine if there are other factors of concern—for example, those unique to OB or surgical patients, or other groups.

The next operational step based on our data is to revise our staffing plan in order to adjust nursing hours per patient day. Our data collection tool allows you to devise your initial plan for revising your staffing plan.

What is a staffing plan?

A staffing plan determines and outlines the number of staff (delineated by job qualification—i.e., RN, LPN, NA, etc.) per department census and budget targets. This plan is utilized for the determination of shift staffing and should be the basis for making decisions related to staffing resources.

To comply with the JCAHO's standards, revising your staffing plan is the most obvious action you should take if there is a correlation between staffing and the clinical indicator under study. Standard HR.2.1 states that the data you collect and analyze must be used to identify potential staffing effectiveness issues and to plan for staffing needs. Thus, creating a staffing plan based on identified needs (incorporating patient satisfaction indicators) is one of the best ways to show that you are planning appropriately for staffing needs. It is important to note, however, that there is a certain amount of subjectivity and "softness" in some measures. In the case of patient satisfaction, it is evident that there are many factors influencing satisfaction besides the sheer number of nurses. Our data do demonstrate, however, that this is a very important factor.

Conclusion: What to do Next

The staffing plan is a "working plan." It incorporates patient census or activity; department activity with staffing variables, such as job qualifications; competence; and patient/staff ratio to delineate staffing resources on a daily basis. Staffing plans should be reviewed dynamically, prior to and midway through each shift, to ensure that appropriate adjustments are made to meet changing needs, facility demands, or increases/decreases in patient census or activity.

A staffing plan must consider and/or incorporate the following:

1. Describe the patient population and the scope of service on the unit
2. Determine how you will assess the acuity of the patients with regard to staffing needs (e.g., patient characteristics that are related to a need for more nursing care)
3. Outline the planned staffing mix for the unit: RNs, LPNs, NAs, and other nonlicensed personnel; perhaps clinical adjunct staff, such as PTs, RTs, social workers, dietitians, etc.; and perhaps members of the staff such as housekeeping. Staffing mix can be expressed as the plan for number of staff per number of patients. See Table 6 below.
4. Footnote hospital standards, benchmarks, and other resources, as well as define the acuity assessment system clearly.

TABLE 6

For example purposes only:

- **Unit:** 10 West Medicine
- **Scope:** General medicine service

Unit census and acuity	Staffing Plan
15-20, no high-acuity patients	Day: 4 RNs, 1 aide, 2 unit sec PM: 3 RNs, 1 aide, 1 unit sec Night: 3 RNs, 1 unit sec
15-20, with 1-3 high acuity patients (based on our hospital's assessment system)	Day: 5 RNs, 1 aide, 2 unit sec PM: 4 RNs, 1 aide, 1 unit sec Night: 3 RNs plus night float among two units, 1 unit sec

Conclusion: What to do Next

The staffing plan should be reviewed periodically—at least annually, in conjunction with budgeting, and more often if there are sentinel events or other critical events that lead management to believe that staffing may be a factor in undesirable outcomes.

The plan should be evaluated formally for its

- ability to deliver desired outcomes (patient satisfaction, clinical measures, etc.)

- budget consistency (similar units perform similarly)

- feasibility (Can we recruit the right number and mix of staff? Or do we have a high rate of vacancies, agency usage, etc.?)

- opportunities for hospital-wide staffing plan improvement—e.g., float staff, flexible assignments, etc.

When JCAHO surveyors review staffing plans and the information used to determine effective staffing, there are several things they will be looking for. Be prepared to demonstrate the following:

- Your planning process for staffing

- The principles you use for staffing: mix of staff, basic ratio you target, and special considerations you would use to adjust the plan

- Your system for assessing the competency of staff, and evidence that it has been implemented (personnel files)

- The rationale for selecting indicators to determine relationships to staffing

- The staff you included in the analysis and staffing plan (direct and indirect care providers)

- Monitoring and aggregating your data over time

- How you evaluate your planning process, and how it indicates improvements or continued modification if improvement is not evident (Show your analysis of variation and your organizational actions. These may be incorporated in your annual unit report, quality report, or even budget.)

Conclusion: What to do Next

- Written evidence of how the staffing effectiveness evaluation and actions are reported to leaders of the organization (This can be incorporated in periodic or annual reports [quality, HR/competency, annual goals, etc.])

Final steps

The final step in the tool is evaluation—determining whether your analysis and intervention were effective, ensuring that you can document this for management and responsible stewardship, and complying with the JCAHO.

As you can see, in our case the final steps after revising your staffing plan are to perform an evaluation and to report to leadership. Part of the evaluation is to determine if your actions have been effective. Once you implement a change based on your data analysis, it is important to continue to measure the indicators over time, as this will help you demonstrate whether there has been improvement. If the data indicate there is no improvement, this is your opportunity to evaluate and adjust actions. Continued measurement is required to track for variation and ensure that actions are still adequate for patient satisfaction and performance improvement. Measurement is key to evaluation, as it demonstrates whether improvement has been effected, and the analysis will serve as a signal to alert us when an undesirable variation occurs. (See the JCAHO PI standards for more discussion of this requirement.)

Conclusion: What to do Next

Post-Intervention Results

Let's jump ahead in time and demonstrate results that you may be able to show as a result of your staffing effectiveness effort.

First, you want to show how you "smoothed" staffing per patient day. By creating a predictable model of approximately 4.5 to 4.7 hours per patient day, hospital-wide (in routine med/surg units), you reduced the fluctuations observed in past data.

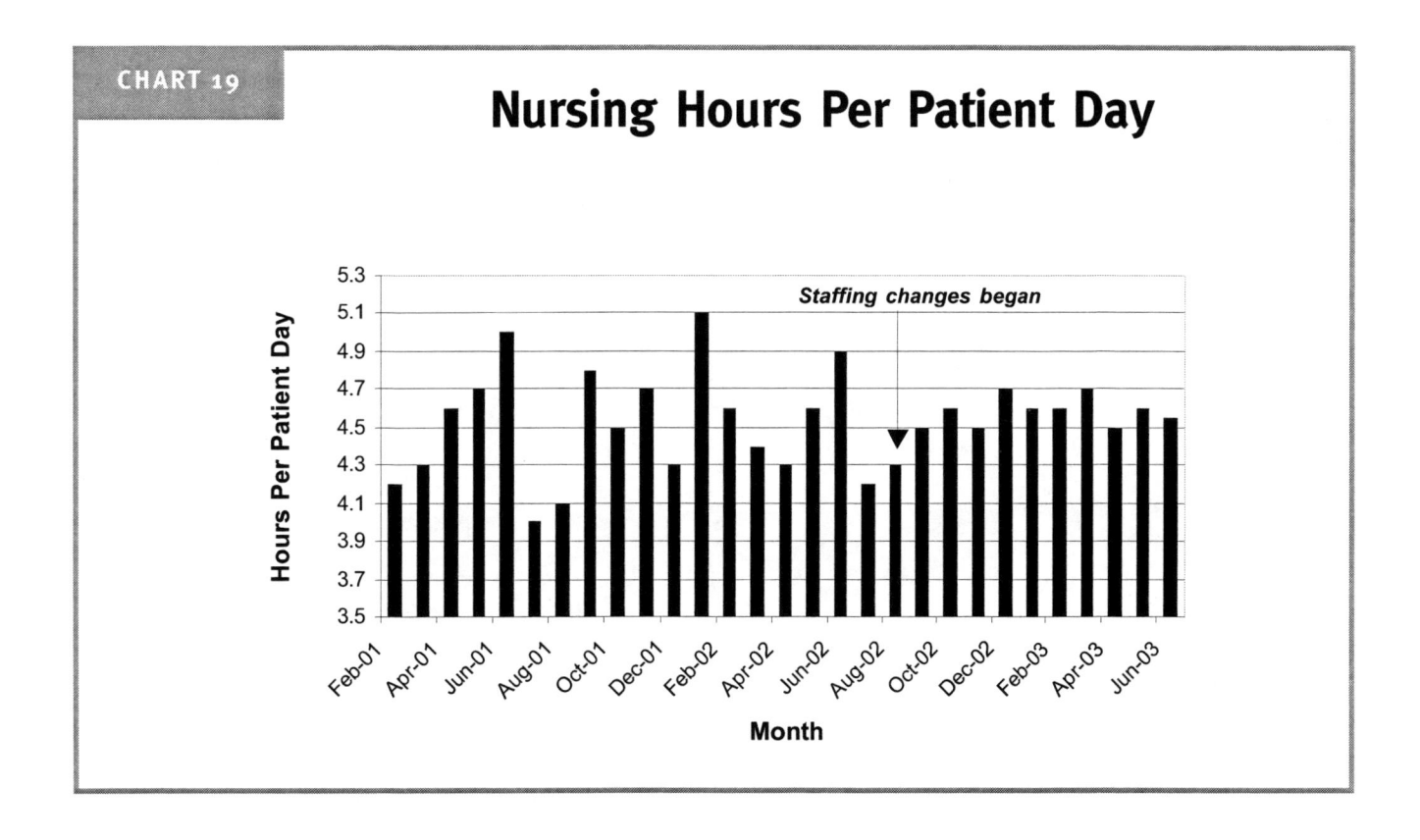

CHART 19

Nursing Hours Per Patient Day

Staffing changes began

CONCLUSION: WHAT TO DO NEXT

Second, you want to verify that the staffing and satisfaction relationship continued to be solid. After reducing the variability in staffing, the absolute level of the correlation was lower, but it was still a clear and strong relationship: Over time, staffing will be more consistent. Now that you have identified the "best" staffing model to accomplish your patient satisfaction goals, if the leadership team follows through, your data will show more and more days and units that are staffing to the "best" level. You should also see that patient satisfaction improves and becomes more consistent. There will be less "variability" in the data and more consistency. This is what you are trying to accomplish.

Note that if you repeat the statistical correlation analysis, however, you will find that this results in a weaker r^2, which is a measure of how much of the variation in patient satisfaction is explained by the variation in nursing hours per patient day. Thus, whatever variation is left in patient satisfaction is less explained by nursing hours per patient day because they aren't varying as much.

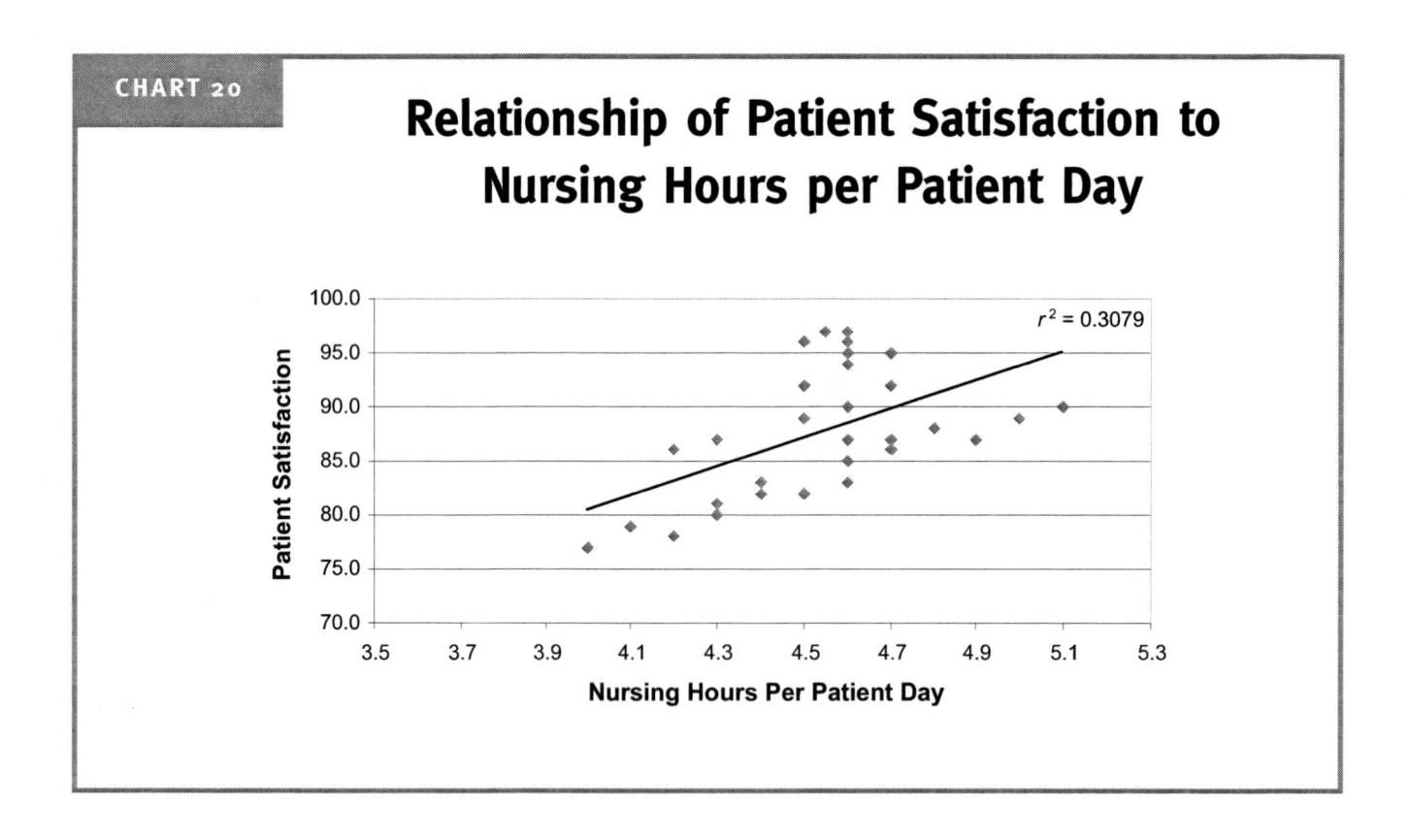

CHART 20

Relationship of Patient Satisfaction to Nursing Hours per Patient Day

$r^2 = 0.3079$

Conclusion: What to do Next

Finally, you want to demonstrate to your oversight committee that, indeed, all of this investment in analysis, intervention, rebudgeting and staff reallocation was effective in improving your key measure: patient satisfaction with nursing care.

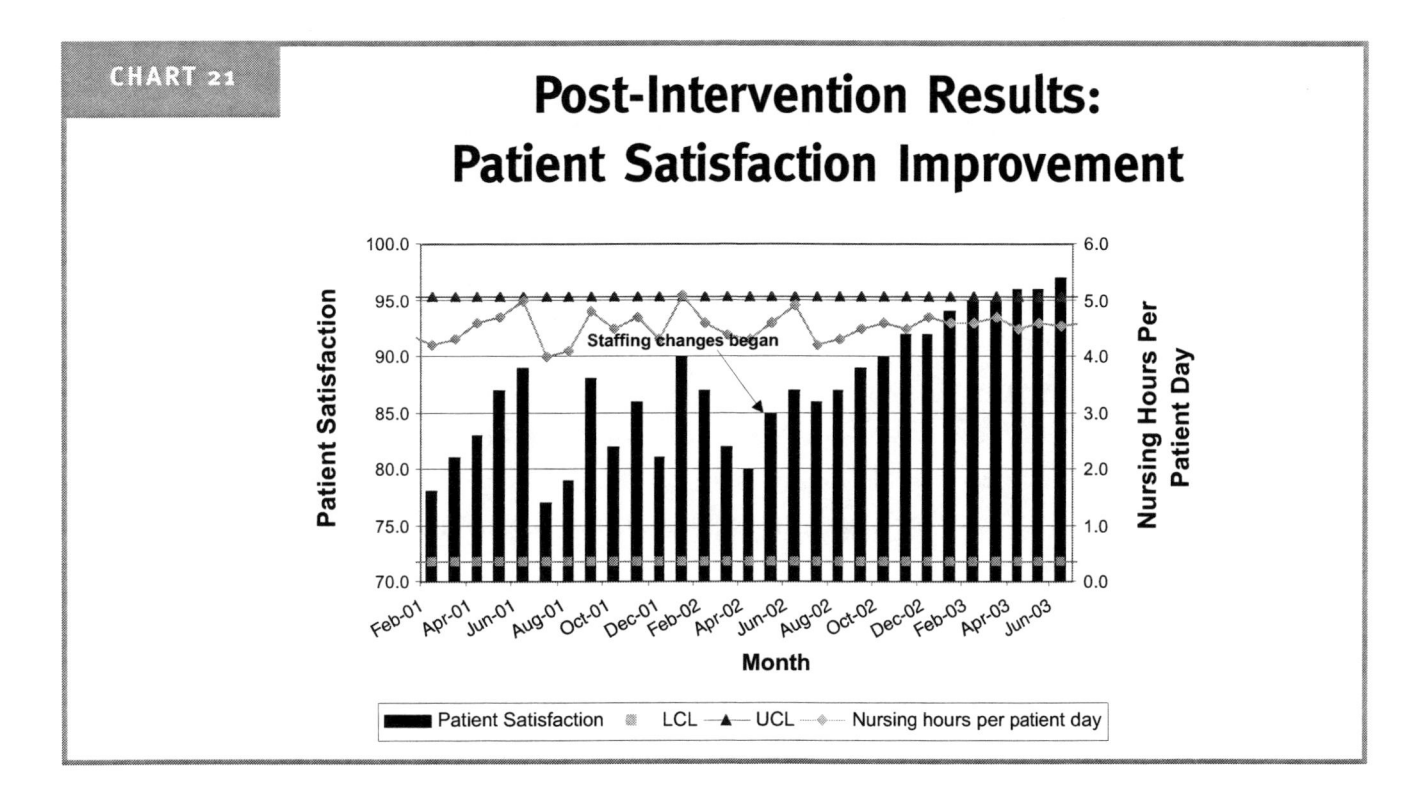

CHART 21

Post-Intervention Results: Patient Satisfaction Improvement

[Bar and line chart showing Patient Satisfaction (bars, left axis 70.0-100.0) and Nursing Hours Per Patient Day (line, right axis 0.0-6.0) from Feb-01 through Jun-03, with an annotation "Staffing changes began" pointing to around mid-2002. Legend: Patient Satisfaction, LCL, UCL, Nursing hours per patient day.]

While complex, chart 21 tells a compelling story.

The "nursing hours per patient day" line is charted on the **right** axis and shows that nurse staffing per patient day has been "smoothed" from its old fluctuations to a more stable and predictable level.

The bars show patient satisfaction levels climbed steadily after the staffing adjustments were implemented, and appear to be holding steady.

The upper and lower control limits demonstrate that the improvement has, indeed, been significant and that the process is now performing statistically differently than it had been previously. You may recall that eight data points above the mean indicate that you have a significant trend. In fact, the mean satisfaction rating across 30 months of data collection is 87%. The 12 satisfaction ratings since July 2002 (August 2002 through July 2003) have all been above the overall mean rating, suggesting that a significant change in satisfaction has occurred.

Conclusion: What to do Next

Not every staffing effectiveness project will be able to tell a story this clear and obvious. The same analytic and presentation techniques will be useful, however, no matter what amount of improvement you can show.

Final considerations

There are two areas we need to consider briefly as we conclude our discussion:

1. Understanding your role in patient satisfaction improvement
2. Demonstrating patient outcomes as they relate to staffing plans

First, the JCAHO expects and requires that leadership and management staff assume responsibility for overall staffing through effective oversight processes and/or direct accountability. It is essential under the JCAHO's standards to **use data as the basis for decision-making**. Data must be used for monitoring trends over time and comparing staffing with your clinical outcomes to ensure both patient satisfaction (and/or other outcomes you have targeted) and effective staffing.

The JCAHO staffing standards extend far beyond the sheer *number* of staff to encompass their recruitment; orientation and training; competency; and ongoing management and coaching. In our case, we focused on a basic and even introductory approach to staffing effectiveness. As your experience with these techniques increases, you can enhance the sophistication of the data you use to assess staffing effectiveness, but you will use the same process regardless of which measures you select.

Second, essential to compliance with the staffing effectiveness standards, you must be able to assess patient outcomes and their relationship to your staffing plans. In our case, it was possible to demonstrate that nursing hours *per patient day* had an influence on patient satisfaction with nursing care. Ultimately, your ability to demonstrate that your staffing plans have been evaluated and are known to be effective in producing the outcomes you targeted will be key to meeting the JCAHO's standards.

The JCAHO's staffing effectiveness standards may seem complex and daunting in their demand for statistical analysis. Like many other regulatory requirements, however, upon careful review it is clear that this is simply a systematic way of evaluating and ensuring that health care organizations are providing safe and effective patient-centered care. The details of this particular standard certainly present some unique challenges, as compared to standards of the past. Full compliance with this standard is well within the reach of every organization, however, and if implemented thoughtfully, it can contribute to a significant improvement in patient care delivery.

Appendix A
Glossary

Appendix A: Glossary

A

adverse drug event: (clinical indicator) harm experienced by a patient due to administration of a medication or failure to administer a medication as planned.

axis: in two dimensions, the span of values along a horizontal line that is placed at a 90-degree angle to the span of values along a vertical line. The axes serve as reference points for data points that appear in graphs.

B

bar chart: a style of data presentation in which categories (for example, patient care units) are plotted along the horizontal axis, and a measure for each of the categories (for example, nursing hours per patient day for each unit) is plotted along the vertical axis. For each x-axis category, a vertical bar will appear whose height is equivalent to the value of the measure for that category (number of nursing hours per patient day for patient care Unit A).

baseline data: a basis of measurement for future use.

C

central tendency: coming to the center; tending toward the middle, typical of a large number of values of a measure.

chi square: statistical method used to determine whether the distribution of one value is contingent upon another value.

clinical or service indicator: measure of patient care outcomes or process/delivery of care.

Appendix A: Glossary

comparison data: the association of information.

correlation coefficient: a statistic that indicates the level of relationship between two measures whose values are paired (such as nursing hours per patient day and patient falls per patient day). It is represented by the letter r, and its values range from -1.0 (negative correlation, indirect relationship) to $+1.0$ (positive correlation, direct relationship). If r equals zero, there is no correlation between the two measures. This can happen either when one of the measures does not vary at all or when the two measures vary but not together.

D

data analysis: the process of studying the information (indicators) or facts collected.

data collection: the process of assembling information or facts for data management to determine the correlation of indicators related to staffing and patient safety.

data measurement: the process of calculating and assessing the information collected.

data range: difference between the largest value and the smallest value.

denominator: for a measure of indicator that is the result of calculating a ratio, the number "on the bottom," which is divided into the numerator.

direct caregivers: staff who provide care directly to patients.

F

family complaints: (clinical indicator) number of complaints received from family members or significant others. Complaints are typically defined as concerns related to patient care and treatment or service. These may involve perceived quality of care, outcome, or costs as well.

H

horizontal bar: a rectangular area on a bar chart the length of which is related to the value a measure (nursing hours per patient day) has for a particular category (patient care Unit A). For example, the rectangular bar might represent 5.2 nursing hours per patient day for patient care Unit A. A bar

Appendix A: Glossary

chart can be presented vertically or horizontally. Your choice of one over the other may relate to the length of labels or the emphasis of the results being presented.

human resource (HR) indicator: measure related to hospital staffing.

I

indirect caregivers: staff who support the provision of care to patients but do not administer patient care directly.

injuries to patients: (clinical indicator) harm of any sort experienced by patients.

L

label: the name of something. In Excel, labels can be associated with the horizontal and vertical axes, as well as the data points that appear in the graph.

length of stay: (clinical indicator) the number of inpatient days per patient (can be computed for each patient or as an aggregate for a group of patients).

line chart: a style of data presentation in which data points are connected by a line. Time is often plotted on the horizontal axis, and you can illustrate trends over time (sometimes referred to as a run chart). If, for example, you have a count of the number of patient complaints on Unit 1 for 12 months, you can present them in a line chart whose horizontal axis is months and whose vertical axis is number of patient complaints.

M

mean: statistic representing the central tendency of multiple observations, it is calculated by adding the values of each observation and dividing by the number of observations.

median: the middle value of a list of numbers. If the list contains an even number of values, the median is half of the sum of the two values closest to the middle in the list. If the list contains an odd number of values, the middle value is the median.

Appendix A: Glossary

N

null hypothesis: the assumption that there is no relationship among variables of interest. (The goal of analysis is to confirm or deny this null hypothesis.)

numerator: for a measure or indicator that is the result of calculating a ratio, the number "on the top," which is divided into the denominator.

numerical variability: the difference in numbers when comparing numerical results.

nursing care hours per patient day: (HR indicator) total number of nursing hours worked, divided by number of patient days of care provided by the hospital or unit of interest.

O

on-call or per-diem use: (HR indicator) these are staff hours utilized to supplement or replace regularly scheduled hours.

overtime hours: (HR indicator) the number of hours worked by staff per shift, day, or month beyond what is allotted for full-time employees.

P

patient complaints: (clinical indicator) number of complaints received from patients.

patient fall: (clinical indicator) an unexpected and actual (not near-miss) descent or lowering to the floor from a bed, chair, or table or while walking, etc.

patient outcome: patient's experience as a result of medical care provided.

Pneumonia (nosocomial): (clinical indicator) patients who acquire pneumonia after admission—not part of the admission diagnosis (utilize the CDC criteria).

postoperative infections: (clinical indicator) the number of patients who develop a postsurgical (Class 1 wound) infection in the inpatient setting or as an outpatient.

APPENDIX A: GLOSSARY

R

r: used to express the correlation coefficient.

ratio: relationship of one measure to another, such as nursing hours per patient days.

rationale: the fundamental reasons for a decision or course of action.

reasonability scan: looking at data, whether subjectively or objectively, to be sure that it makes sense and relates to real world experience.

regression equation: a mathematical formula that describes the expected relationship between two or more measures based on the patterns of historical values of the measures.

S

screening indicator: a defined topic for measurement.

shock/cardiac arrest: (clinical indicator) any patient who experiences loss of pulse or respiration, or a significant deterioration in core vital signs that requires immediate intervention to prevent cardiac or respiratory arrest (typically excludes DNR-status patients).

sick time: (HR indicator) unscheduled or previously unplanned time off.

skin breakdown: (clinical indicator) any incident of skin breakdown that occurs after a patient's admission.

staff injuries on the job: (HR indicator) any reportable injuries that cause harm to staff personnel during working hours.

staff satisfaction: (HR indicator) varies depending on methodology. For example, it may be the number of satisfied staff divided by the number of total staff.

staff turnover rate: (HR indicator) varies depending on organization. For example, the total number of staff departures from any position for any reason divided by total number of employed staff during the period.

Appendix A: Glossary

staff vacancy rate: (HR indicator) the number of unfilled positions divided by the number of total budgeted positions.

staffing effectiveness: the number, competency, and skill mix of staff, as related to the provision of needed services (as defined by the JCAHO).

staffing effectiveness standards: the standards defined by JCAHO, incorporating HR.2.1, PI.3.1, PI.3.1.1, PI.4.3, and LD.4.3.

staffing plan: a plan that determines the number and skill mix of staff (delineated by job qualification—i.e., RN, LPN, NA, etc.) per department census and budget targets.

standard deviation: a statistic, calculated from a list of values, that indicates the level of variability in the values on the list. If all the values are the same, there is no variability and the standard deviation is zero. If the values are very different from one another, the standard deviation is large. A rule of thumb is that you will lose statistical validity in your analysis when the standard deviation is half as large as the mean of the list of values.

standardized: made comparable, adjusted for bias, set on a "level playing field," reduced to a common denominator, tending to be alike.

statistical correlation: statistical method used to determine if there is a relationship between two measures.

statistical variance: statistic calculated to represent numerical spread. See discussion under numerical variance.

strength of relationship: the extent to which two measures vary together, whether positively (direct relationship) or negatively (inverse relationship). *r* values that approach −1.0 or +1.0 demonstrate a strong relationship; those approaching zero demonstrate a weak relationship.

T

t-test: statistical method used to determine whether two group measures are different.

APPENDIX A: GLOSSARY

time period: specified duration over which measures making up HR and/or clinical indicators are gathered for examining relationship; span of time over which each data point (HR or clinical) is collected; used for run charts, reviewing trends, and evaluating performance improvement.

U

understaffing as compared to organization's staffing plan: (HR indicator) the number of positions not staffed in accordance with the staffing plan.

upper gastrointestinal (GI) bleeding: (clinical indicator) the number of patients who develop an acute onset of upper GI bleeding after admission and whose admission symptoms were not GI related.

urinary tract infections (UTIs): (clinical indicator) the number of patients who develop UTIs in the inpatient setting, not as a part of the admitting diagnosis.

V

variation: a deviation or difference; something different from another.

vertical bar: a rectangular area on a bar chart the height of which is related to the value a measure (patient complaints per patient day) has for a particular category (patient care unit A). For example, the bar might reflect three patient complaints per patient day in patient care Unit A. A bar chart can be presented vertically or horizontally. Your choice of one over the other may relate to length of labels or emphasis of results being presented.

X

x-y plot: a style of data presentation in which the horizontal axis represents ranges of values of one measure (number of patient falls per month), and the vertical axis represents ranges of values of another measure (number of nursing hours per patient day). Values of pairs of the measures become a data point in the chart. The x-y plot is a visual representation of the relationship between the two measures. It is common to show the "independent" or "causing" variable on the horizontal axis and the "dependent" or "result" variable on the vertical axis.

Appendix B
Tools

Appendix B: Tools

Quality Improvement Planning and Monitoring Tool

Enter Hospital Name

Quality Improvement Planning and Monitoring	Date:

PROCESS: Staffing Effectiveness

Overview, History, Why Important:
(Describe the pair of measures used to assess staffing effectiveness, why selected, hypothesis.)

Performance Dimensions and Goals:
(Describe the goal of the analysis: link these measures through correlation and other analyses to assess possible improvements in staff to improve outcome.)

Current Period Performance:
(Relevant data in graphic and/or tabular format [here or attached].)

Trend: Performance Over Time:
(Relevant data in graphic and/or tabular format [here or attached].)

FINDINGS AND CONCLUSIONS

Are the measures linked? What evidence of statistical relationship do you have?

Is staffing effective to achieve the desired outcome at this time? How do you know?

If not, what are team conclusions about potential areas for improvement?

What additional data, pilot studies, small-scale tests of change, etc. are needed?

STRATEGIES: Recommendations to be implemented/referred for action

Action *Including attention to new opportunities for improvement*	**By Whom**	**By When**

FOLLOW UP

Date:

Review data again

Update on referred recommendations

Report at unit/department meeting

Report to medical director/clinical leadership

Approved: _____

APPENDIX B: TOOLS

Staffing Effectiveness Data Plan Tool

HOSPITAL NAME
Quality Improvement Planning and Monitoring

STAFFING EFFECTIVENESS DATA PLAN

Name of measure set:

Inpatient care areas/patient populations *(describe population)*:

Types of practitioners/workers/providers *(describe practioners)*:

Indicator Pairs: *Enter indicator pairs (e.g., nursing hours and patient satisfaction)*

Staffing Effectiveness Measure Set 1 (*define hypothesis or area to explore*):

1a. HR INDICATOR

Why important *(check one or more)*:	High Volume	High Risk	Problem Prone	Other Criteria
Selected from JCAHO list or hospital specific:	JCAHO list		Hospital-specific	
Caregivers *(check either or both)*:	Direct		Indirect	

Clearly define numerator or data element:

Clearly define denominator as relevant:

Sample: (define: 100% or sample):

Methodology (e.g., chart review, abstract from computerized reports):

Source (e.g., medical record, personnel system, surveys):

Benchmark, if any (source of external comparative data):

Frequency (monthly, quarterly, weekly, etc.)

1b. CLINICAL/SERVICE INDICATOR

Why important *(check one or more:)*:	High Volume	High Risk	Problem Prone	Other Criteria

Clearly define denominator as relevant:

Sample: (define: 100% or sample):

Methodology (e.g., chart review, abstract from computerized reports):

Source (e.g., medical record, personnel system, surveys):

Benchmark, if any (source of external comparative data):

Frequency (monthly, quarterly, weekly, etc.)

Staffing Effectiveness Data Plan Tool (cont.)

2a. HR INDICATOR

Why important (check one or more:)	High Volume	High Risk	Problem Prone	Other Criteria
Selected from JCAHO list or hospital specific:	JCAHO list		Hospital-specific	
Caregivers: direct, indirect (check either or both)	Direct		Indirect	

Clearly define numerator or data element:

Clearly define denominator as relevant:

Sample: (define: 100% or sample):

Methodology (e.g., chart review, abstract from computerized reports):

Source (e.g., medical record, personnel system, surveys):

Benchmark, if any (source of external comparative data):

Frequency (monthly, quarterly, weekly, etc.)

2b. CLINICAL/SERVICE INDICATOR

Why important (check one or more:)	High Volume	High Risk	Problem Prone	Other Criteria

Clearly define denominator as relevant:

Sample: (define: 100% or sample):

Methodology (e.g., chart review, abstract from computerized reports):

Source (e.g., medical record, personnel system, surveys):

Benchmark, if any (source of external comparative data):

Frequency (monthly, quarterly, weekly, etc.)

Analysis plan (*describe briefly*):

Unit of measure (hospital wide, department, etc) (*describe briefly*):

Date Updated:_____

Approved By:_____